BATH BOMBS, BODY SCRUBS & MORE!

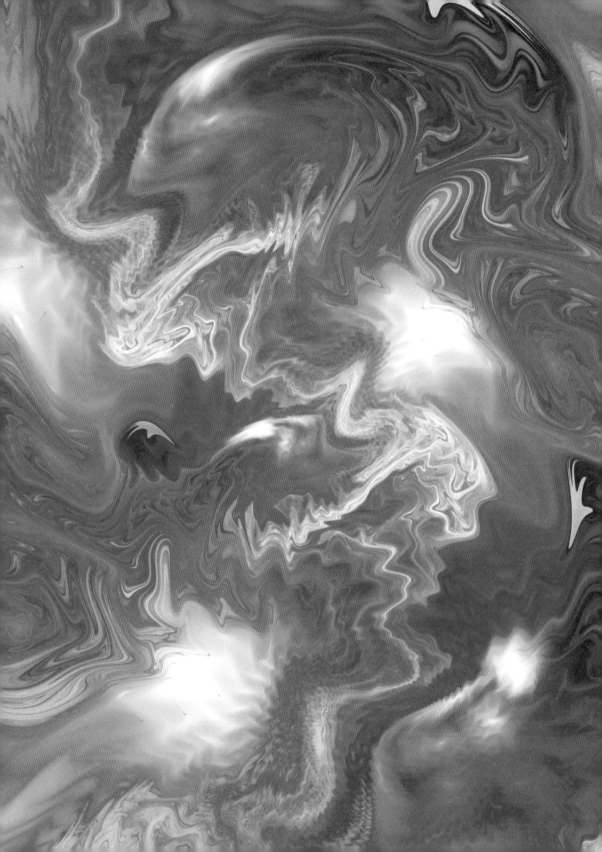

BATH BOMBS, BODY SCRUBS & MORE!

OVER 50 NATURAL BATH AND BEAUTY RECIPES FOR GORGEOUS SKIN

ISABEL BERCAW &
CAROLINE BERCAW

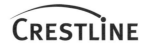

© 2018 by Quarto Publishing Group USA Inc.

Da Bomb is a registered trademark of Da Bomb, LLC.

"Sisterpreneurs" is a trademark of Da Bomb, LLC.

This edition published in 2019 by Crestline, an imprint of The Quarto Group
142 West 36th Street, 4th Floor
New York, NY 10018 USA
T (212) 779-4972 **F** (212) 779-6058
www.QuartoKnows.com

First published in 2018 by Rock Point, an imprint of The Quarto Group
142 West 36th Street, 4th Floor
New York, NY 10018 USA.

Crestline titles are also available at discount for retail, wholesale, promotional, and bulk purchase. For details, contact the Special Sales Manager by email at specialsales@quarto.com or by mail at The Quarto Group, Attn: Special Sales Manager, 100 Cummings Center Suite 265D, Beverly, MA 01915, USA.

Previously published as Fizz Boom Bath: Learn to Make Your Own Bath Bombs, Body Scrubs, and More!

10 9 8 7 6 5 4 3 2 1

ISBN: 978-0-7858-3730-5

Photography: Evi Abeler
Editorial Director: Rage Kindelsperger
Creative Director: Merideth Harte
Managing Editor: Erin Canning
Editor: John Foster
Cover Designer: Philip Buchanan
Interior Design: Tara Long

Printed in China

This book provides general information on various widely known and widely accepted images that tend to evoke feelings of strength and confidence. However, it should not be relied upon as recommending or promoting any specific diagnosis or method of treatment for a particular condition, and it is not intended as a substitute for medical advice or for direct diagnosis and treatment of a medical condition by a qualified physician. Readers who have questions about a particular condition, possible treatments for that condition, or possible reactions from the condition or its treatment should consult a physician or other qualified healthcare professional.

Common Sense Warnings:
We know they look and smell amazing, but the bath and body products in this book are not edible. Some make your tub slippery, so be careful. Avoid contact with eyes and mouth. Avoid use if your skin is cracked or damaged, and always test on a small area of skin before initial use. Suitable for people over the age of three.

To Mom and Dad: Now that we're published authors, can we stay out past midnight?

CONTENTS

Introduction
1

Materials
7

Ingredients
8

Equipment
13

15
Part One: Bath Bombs

How to Make a Bath Bomb
16

Fruity Fragrances
19

Nutty + Spicy Fragrances
39

Floral Fragrances
51

Aromatherapy Fragrances
63

77
Part Two: More Bath + Beauty Products

Face, Lips + Hair
79

Soaks + Melts
99

Hands, Feet + Everything Else
111

Afterword
130

Resources
131

Acknowledgments
132

About the Authors
133

Index
134

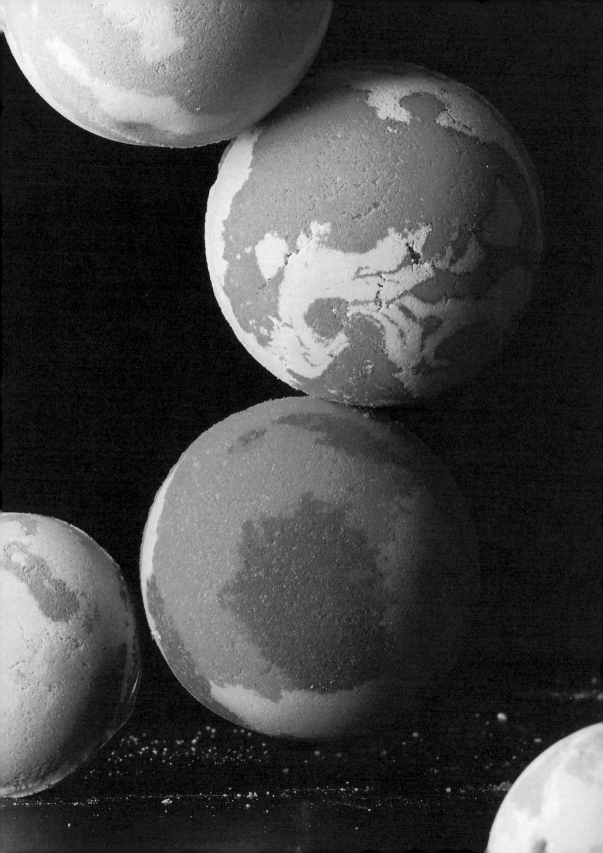

INTRODUCTION

HAVE YOU EVER BEEN at a store and found yourself staring longingly at a table full of gorgeous-looking bath bombs, shower melts, or lotion bars and thought, "Hey, it would be fun to make these at home, but where the heck would I begin?" Well, we're here to take the mystery out of bath and body recipes and give you all the tools you need to crown yourself the Archbishop of Bathtopia. We'll hold your hand every step of the way, and then we'll exfoliate it with some sugar scrub when we're finished! This book will teach you how to create all kinds of natural, homemade treats. From fizzers to scrubs, bubble bars to lip balm, we've got you covered. And why should you take advice from a couple of teenage sisters, you may ask? Before we get to the good stuff, we should probably explain who we are and how we came to write this book.

SIS BOOM BATH

It was December of 2012. We were ten and twelve years old, it was winter break, and we were bored. (Snapchat did not yet exist; you get it.) We had always loved using fizzing bath bombs, but there were a few big problems with the ones we bought

at the mall. First of all, each one contained over a dozen ingredients, most of which we couldn't pronounce. They also had heavy, greasy additives that left our tub full of gunk and made us feel dirtier after our baths than when we started. And when a bomb finished dissolving and we drained the tub, we were usually left with sticky substances like seaweed,

WE'RE HERE TO TAKE THE MYSTERY OUT OF BATH AND BODY RECIPES AND GIVE YOU ALL THE TOOLS YOU NEED

often mixed with a foamy muck that stuck to our skin and made us feel like something out of *Stranger Things*. We would usually have to take a shower after each bath to get clean! But we still loved the idea of a fun, fizzing sphere that filled the room with amazing fragrances and the bath with just enough (but not too many) moisturizing oils.

So it seemed like a good idea to try and make our own bath bombs. We hit the internet, looked for the least complicated recipe we could

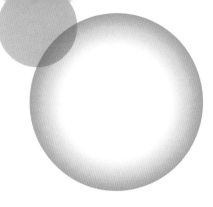

find, and then came up with the wild idea of putting a little surprise in each bath bomb so we'd have something fun left at the end. We found most of the ingredients we needed at our local grocery store, except for the citric acid, which our mom helped us order online. We scoured the kitchen for measuring cups and mixing bowls, arranged them on an old blanket in our basement, and waited excitedly for our citric acid to arrive so we could begin our grand experiment. (For all the ingredients *you'll* need to make bath bombs and more, see pages 8–13.)

Once all our ingredients and supplies were in place, we spent an entire afternoon carefully strategizing, reading, measuring, mixing, and

SOON, OUR FRIENDS WERE ASKING IF THEY COULD USE OUR PRODUCTS, SO WE GAVE THEM AWAY TO ANYONE WHO WOULD TRY THEM.

molding, and when the dust cleared (yes, making bath bombs is dusty), we had seven and a half lopsided, lumpy, crumbly, half fizzed-out bath bombs. We were pretty proud of ourselves.

The only thing more exciting than making those bath bombs was using them. After we let them dry overnight, we won the award for Earliest Bath Ever by hopping in the tub at 6:00 a.m., because we just *had* to see if our efforts would pay off. You can probably imagine how psyched we were when our cracked, oddball creations fizzed away under the warm water of our bath, releasing a lavender fragrance and turning the water a pretty blue. With that first, fateful experiment, we were hooked.

Over the next several months, we spent our free time testing out new bath bomb recipes, botching plenty of batches, trying out all kinds of color combos, and even moving on to other bath and body treats like sugar scrubs, salt soaks, and face masks. We had a whole room in the basement to ourselves, and our parents had only one solid rule: Whatever mess you make, clean it up. Soon, our friends were asking if they could use our products, so we gave them away to anyone who would try them. We even sold some to our grandma! Not too long after that, our friend Dialyn encouraged us to sign up for a local art fair that had a special section for kids. It cost about $25 for a table—which to us was a life's savings at the time—but we figured, "Why not?"

We decided to focus on bath bombs and spent all summer making about 150 of them in preparation for the art fair. We gave each bath bomb its own name, color, and fragrance and put a surprise inside. The Cake Bomb was white with rainbow-colored sprinkles, had an almond buttercream fragrance, and contained an eraser shaped like a piece of cake. We made a red Cherry Bomb that smelled like maraschino cherries and had a little plastic cherry inside. We made an "F" Bomb that smelled like lavender and contained a calming message. (Our parents vetoed that one immediately, but we convinced them the F stood for *frustration*, and the "F" Bomb calms your frustrations. They reluctantly let us include it in our product line.) One of our favorites was—and still is—the Earth Bomb, which has blue, green, and white swirls, smells like a sea breeze, and has a cute little toy ocean creature inside. We decided to donate some of the money from the sale of the Earth Bomb to organizations that clean up the world's oceans. (Today, the Earth Bomb is our top seller and we've donated tens of thousands of dollars to the cause.)

Originally, we molded our bath bombs using a snowball maker we found lying around the house. We decided to pile our bath bombs into black, gallon-sized plastic buckets purchased at the dollar store, and we planned to display them unpackaged, so people could pick them up and smell them. Each time we made a sale, we would carefully place each bomb in a clear cellophane bag and tie it with a black ribbon. The finishing touch was a tag featuring the name of the bomb and our brand name: Da Bomb Bath Fizzers.

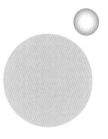

We were really nervous on the first day of the art fair. Would anyone want to buy our products? Would all of our hard work pay off? Or would we have to drag this 840-pound load of bath bombs back to our house at the end of the day?

To our utter amazement, before we even finished setting up our table, people started crowding around, asking lots of questions, and buying our products. Our idea of setting the bombs out unpackaged worked great, because the fragrances filled the air around our table, and people flocked to see what smelled so good. By the end of the day we were exhausted, and we had sold out! We couldn't believe it.

Despite our success, we still didn't think of Da Bomb as anything other than a hobby. When the art fair rolled around the following year, we decided to participate again. At one point during that second fair, a local salon owner named Mitchell Wherley stopped by and purchased a few

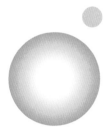

of our bath bombs. The following day, he visited us again, bought a dozen more bombs, and asked us if he could sell our products in his salons! We suddenly realized our hobby had the potential to become

ORDERS BEGAN ROLLING IN SO QUICKLY WE COULDN'T KEEP UP

a real business. Not only did he place an order, he placed a reorder. And another. And another. Then a second local retailer requested our bath bombs. And everyone kept asking if we had a website. So, with a lot of help from our parents, we created our very own website in April of 2015: DaBombFizzers.com. Then, we officially became Da Bomb, LLC.

BECOMING SISTERPRENEURS™
Over the next several months, we did more art fairs and events and even appeared on the local news a few times. Word started to spread about the young sisters who make bath bombs with surprises inside. Orders began rolling in so quickly we couldn't keep up, so our mom started helping us make the bombs. But soon, her help wasn't enough and we asked our

dad to jump in, too. One day, we all looked at each other and realized we either needed to pull the plug on this crazy adventure or dive in all the way. (You already know what we decided.) Shortly after that, we hired our first official employee, Miguel. He agreed to come to our house almost every night for several hours and make the bombs for us while our family focused on filling and shipping orders.

By that time, we had made a small amount of money to reinvest in the business, and we decided to spend it on better packaging. We came up with some really cool ideas, and with the help of a local designer and printing company, we were able to create packaging that was eye-popping and totally unique. Our sales began to soar.

By October 2015, we had eight employees working out of our house. It was then that both of our parents decided to work full time for the business. Our dad closed the doors on his small management consulting company and our mom decided to put her advertising writing experience to good use by helping us perfect our brand identity. Together, our parents' skill sets gave us just the support we needed to push Da Bomb Bath Fizzers onward and upward.

With everyone's help, we were now making and selling 20,000 bath bombs a month! It was a crazy time. There were bath bombs everywhere— in our kitchen, our family room, upstairs, downstairs. Our living room was the shipping department. Our finished attic was where the bombs went to dry. And our neighbors could smell our bath bomb fragrances all the way down the street. We officially needed a commercial location. After four months of careful searching, we found just the right place for Da Bomb headquarters. It was a small, recently finished office space attached to a four-thousand-square-foot warehouse where we could continue to make our bombs and grow our business. The best part? It was just a few miles from our house. Along with our parents, we made the decision to sign a five-year lease, and much to our surprise, within two months we were contacting the property owner to see if we could expand to the warehouse

next door! We continued to add wholesale accounts, including some large retailers like Target and Hy-Vee grocery stores. We even went to our first trade show and gained a ton of new wholesale accounts. People really responded to our story, our packaging was unlike anything else on the market, and everyone loved the fact that our bath bombs had surprises inside. It was a trifecta of awesomeness.

Fast-forward to today. Our products are now in thousands of stores. We employ more than 150 people in our community. And now we even get to write our own book! And if our ten- and twelve-year-old selves were able to figure out how to make bath and body products at home, we're pretty sure you can, too. So are you ready? Let's make some bath treats!

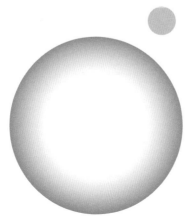

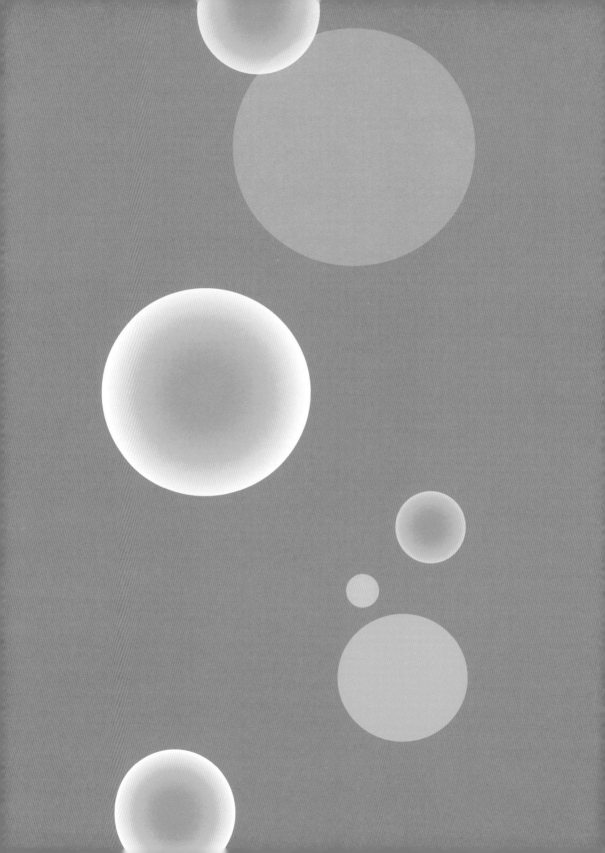

MATERIALS

OKAY, THIS IS THE PART WHERE YOU FIGURE
OUT WHAT YOU HAVE, WHAT YOU NEED,
AND WHAT TO MAKE FIRST! WE SUGGEST
ASSESSING WHAT SUPPLIES ARE CURRENTLY
AT YOUR DISPOSAL AND PICKING YOUR
FIRST RECIPE BASED ON THEM. OR IF YOU'RE
ONE OF THOSE PATIENT, METHODICAL TYPES,
YOU'LL PROBABLY WANT TO STUDY
THIS BOOK FROM COVER TO COVER!

INGREDIENTS

To make the bath bombs and beauty products in this book, you'll need some specific ingredients and equipment. Some of these items are things that you might already have around the house, and others need to be bought or ordered from specialty stores. Check the resources section at the end of the book for where to buy some of the harder-to-find items. And don't be afraid to experiment a little. Some of the best results happen when you think you've botched something. (Have we told you about the time we invented bath bomb crumbles?)

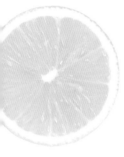

BAKING SUPPLIES

Lots of the recipes in this book use standard baking supplies you may already have in your kitchen. Sugar gives exfoliating power to scrubs, while baking soda (when combined with citric acid) provides the necessary chemical reaction to make your bath bombs fizz.

FRUITS, VEGETABLES, AND OTHER FOOD

Fruits, like strawberries and lemons, and vegetables, like avocados and cucumbers, form the base of many of the non–bath bomb items in this book. These all-natural ingredients offer skin-refreshing citric acid, vitamins, and other good-for-you elements. Hair and face masks, made to moisturize and strengthen, often contain ingredients packed with protein like milk and eggs.

COCONUT OIL, SWEET ALMOND OIL, AND MORE

Most of the products in this book use coconut oil and sweet almond oil, which are clear, long-lasting oils with very little fragrance. When purchasing coconut oil, look for fractionated coconut oil, which is a liquid—as opposed to regular coconut oil, which is usually solid at room temperature and can be harder to work with. You can also experiment with other widely available oils; for example, we use apricot oil and chia seed oil pretty regularly. You can even use olive oil, grapeseed oil, or other cooking oils, but they tend to go bad within a few months and might give you weird colors (bath bombs may even start to discolor after a few weeks).

CITRIC ACID

When combined with baking soda, citric acid gives bath bombs their awesome fizzy properties. You can find it online—check the resources section for some options.

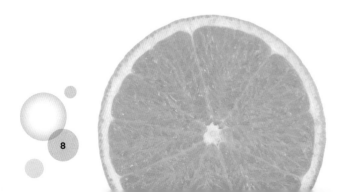

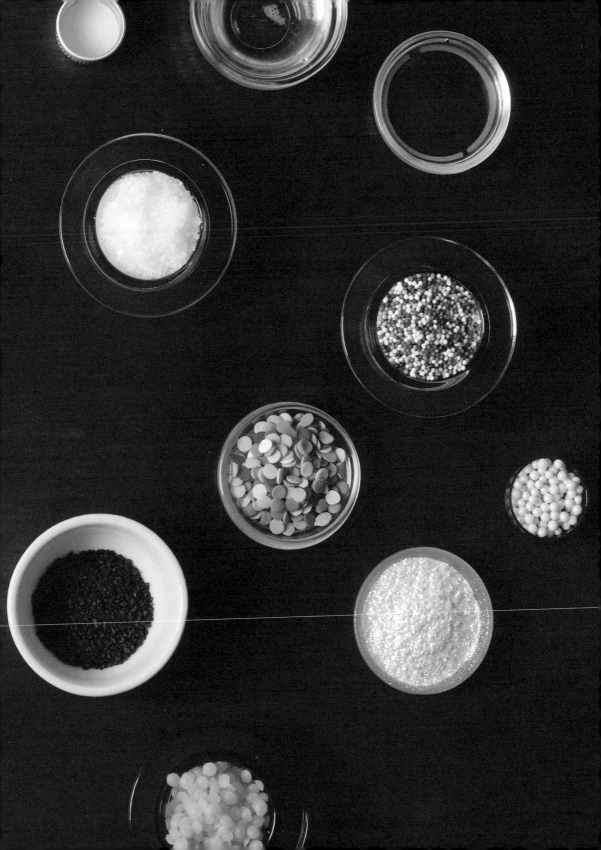

VITAMIN E OIL

Vitamin E oil is great to add to beauty products because it nourishes your skin and is a preservative, helping the product last longer. Look for it at a health-food store or online. If you can't find a bottle with a dropper, you can also buy vitamin E capsules and break them open. Make sure to buy the kind labeled "real," not "synthetic."

FRAGRANCE OILS AND ESSENTIAL OILS

Bath bombs aren't bath bombs without their wonderful fragrances, and we've given you a lot of combinations to try out in the following pages. We prefer using fragrance oils instead of essential oils because they last longer, but some people feel that essential oils have more healing benefits. Whether you choose to use essential oils or fragrance oils, be sure to purchase them from a reputable source. Both types of oils can irritate sensitive skin if not diluted properly. As with any product that comes in direct contact with your skin, always test it on a small part of your body before "diving in," especially if it's the first time you've used a particular product.

BUTTERS

Butters help firm up products like lotion, lip balms, and body bars. We like to use cocoa butter, mango butter, and coffee butter, but you can experiment with all different kinds of butters, like avocado and shea, and substitute them when butters are recommended.

BEESWAX

Beeswax is another ingredient that's used to firm up products like lotion bars and balms. It's hard—and can be hard to break up—so make sure to get beeswax pellets rather than a block. You should also look for beeswax labeled "cosmetic grade."

COLORING

There are lots of ways to add color to your bath and body products. Some people prefer subtle, pastel hues, while others love bright, bold pigments. See the resources section for a few sources. For more brightly colored bombs, increase the amount of color as desired.

Keep in mind that any time you use a pigment, there's a possibility that the color could stain your bath, your skin, or both. Factors that may affect staining include the age of your bathtub, what material the tub is made of, and even how much water you put into the bath. While traditional food coloring is commonly used in homemade bath bomb and bath products, we recommend liquid colors formulated specifically for this purpose. These are safer for your bathtub and your skin. Using them means you can enjoy a blue bath bomb without looking like a Smurf for two days afterward. But when in doubt, start out using less pigment and work your way up.

HINT: If you don't want to mess with dividing your bath bomb batch in order to create multiple colors of mix, you can simplify the recipe by making a full batch of each color! $1/2$ teaspoon of liquid color per batch should be adequate.

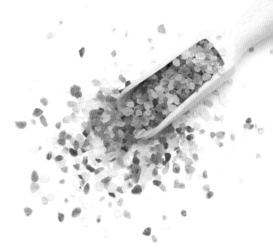

WITCH HAZEL AND EPSOM SALTS

Witch hazel is an astringent used to tighten your pores. Epsom salts are used in some of the bath salts and soaks; they are full of magnesium, which is great for sore muscles. Although you may have never heard of either of these products, you can usually find both in the beauty section of your local drugstore.

DECORATIONS AND EMBELLISHMENTS

Part of what makes our bath bombs so much fun is the way we decorate them and put surprises inside. We've given you some suggestions on how to create your own "surprise" bombs. From candy sprinkles to dried flowers to messages, don't be afraid to get creative!

MICA POWDER AND ECO GLITTER

Craving something extra? Sparkling mica powder will give your creations that elevated level of awesomeness you desire. You'll find several online suppliers of these listed in the resources section. "Eco Glitter" is always a good bet, as well, because it is 100 percent biodegradable and safe for your pipes. Steer clear of traditional glitter, which is bad for the environment and can stick to your skin.

PRODUCTS TO MAKE BUBBLES (AKA SURFACTANTS)

A few of the products in the book just meant to be bubbly. Bubbles are made with a chemical called a surfactant, and there are dozens of different types. Because surfactants, on rare occasions, may irritate some people's skin, we've included the gentlest options we could find. To make it simple, we've given you directions using a clear liquid-soap base. This can simply be a shower gel or hand soap you get at a drugstore, or it can be a clear liquid-soap base you buy from one of the places listed in the Resources section on page 131. (By using a clear liquid-soap base, which is fragrance-free, you have the option of adding whatever fragrance you want.) As you become more experienced making bath products from scratch, you might want to experiment with using sodium laureth sulfate, or SLES. Although we don't include instructions for using it in this book, you can find instructions online that explain how using SLES allows you to have more control over the amount of bubbles, as well as the other ingredients in your product. SLES comes in powder form and is less harsh than its better-known cousin, sodium lauryl sulfate (SLS). You can buy SLES from one of the sources in the Resources section as well. Lathanol (LAL) is another powder that will produce bubbles and is worth experimenting with. It's even milder than SLES, which will make your skin happy, but it produces smaller bubbles.

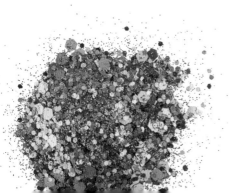

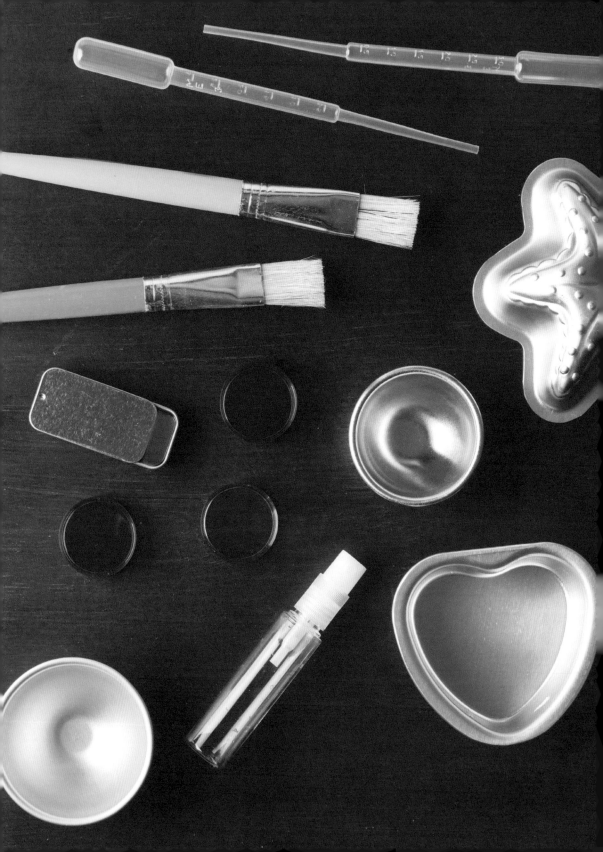

EQUIPMENT

Pretty much every time we dive into a new project, we end up having the most fun during the planning phase. What supplies will we use? Will we need to purchase something new, or can we use what's already on hand in a creative way? (As we mentioned in the introduction, when we first started making bath bombs, we used a plastic snowball maker to mold them!) And how long will it take our mom to figure out we raided the utensil drawer? Nothing beats that lightning bolt moment when a great idea sparks. Think of this section of the book your formal invitation to channel your inner hunter-gatherer and scour your home for some useful materials!

BOWLS AND OTHER CONTAINERS

Head to the kitchen and grab some small and medium mixing bowls. You'll need them to mix together various products. In many cases, you'll also need a container to store the finished product. For masks and scrubs, you can just use plastic containers with lids, like Tupperware. But you may want nicer (glass) containers if you're giving your creations as gifts or if you just want to pamper yourself. For items like lip balms, you may need to buy small containers, like empty lip balm tubes, online to pour the hot balm in to harden. For sprays, search online for empty atomizer (spray) bottles.

PAINTBRUSHES

When using mica powder to make your bath bombs extra sparkly, you'll need a paintbrush to paint it on.

PIPETTES

Pipettes are liquid droppers. They're used for transferring some hot homemade beauty products (like lotion bars before they've hardened) into molds and are essential for adding oils and other products to your creations when they don't come with droppers. They're also great for stirring, because you can throw them away and don't have to worry about the product hardening on your kitchen utensils.

MOLDS

Molds are vital for making solid bath bombs as well as other solid bath products like bath jellies and lotion bars. They come in a variety of shapes, sizes, and materials. We recommend reusable rubber or metal molds for bath bombs and rubber for lotion bars. Unless otherwise noted, the sphere-shaped bath bombs in this book were made with tennis ball–sized molds approximately 2.75 inches (7 cm) in diameter. This size will yield 3 to 4 bombs in a batch. As usual, we think experimenting with different shapes is part of the fun, but we've also given you some different examples throughout using just about every shape of mold we could find. Don't hesitate to look around your house for items you might have on hand that could work well. Kitchen staples like cookie cutters, muffin pans, and even small measuring cups can make great molds!

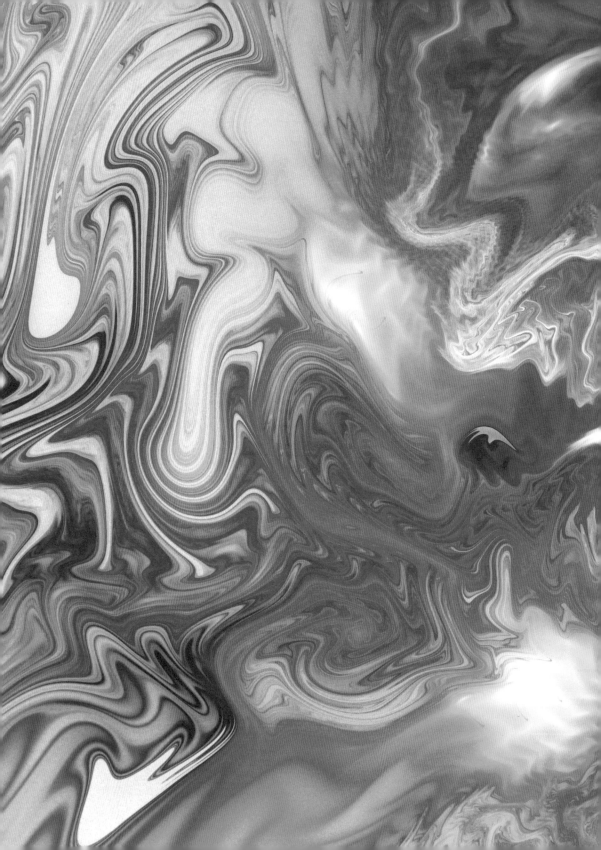

PART ONE

· · · · · · · · · · · · · · · ·

BATH
BOMBS

HOW TO MAKE A BATH BOMB

MAKES 3-4 BOMBS

OKAY, PEOPLE. THIS ISN'T ROCKET SCIENCE, but there *is* chemistry involved and it never hurts to understand the basics. The two main ingredients in a bath bomb are baking soda and citric acid. When you mix them together and combine them with water, carbon dioxide gas is released, hence the "fizz." This is called an acid-base reaction, and it's pretty fun to watch. To make the bomb stick together, most people use what's called a "binding agent." Our binding agent of choice is oil. We also include cornstarch in our recipe, because it's a natural water softener and the color and fragrance are fun bonuses! Though there's virtually no limit to the ingredients you can add—think kaolin clay, cocoa butter, shea butter, Epsom salts—we like to keep it simple. Below is an easy, basic bath bomb recipe that you can use as a starting point. Part of what we find so much fun about making bath bombs is experimenting with different fragrances, shapes, color combos, and even oils—so feel free to switch things up and don't be afraid to end up with a few misshapen or crumbling bombs that are just . . . bombs. That's part of the fun! For dozens of specific ideas and recipes, see the following pages.

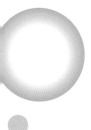

1 In a large bowl, mix together the baking soda, citric acid, and cornstarch.

2 In a separate bowl, combine the oil, fragrance, and liquid color.

3 Add the wet ingredients to the dry ingredients and mix with your hands until the mixture becomes the consistency of wet sand. (If you don't like to get your hands messy, you can wear rubber gloves for this part.) The more vigorous your mixing style, the better the ingredients will be distributed, so don't be shy.

4 Five minutes of stirring, compressing, and kneading should do the trick.

5 Next, press the mixture firmly into your molds, and then let the bombs dry for about 24–48 hours. (It sometimes takes more or less time, depending on the temperature and humidity of the air.)

TIP: If you're using a mold with two halves and the halves aren't sticking together, try overfilling each half before pressing the pieces together firmly. If the mold is spherical, you can also twist the halves back and forth slightly as you press them together for a nice, well-formed shape.

6 Once they are completely dry, remove them carefully from the molds. If you only have one mold, you can also gently remove the bombs as you make them and lay them out to dry on a flat surface. Try not to touch them until they harden.

7 Once they're ready, the real fun begins. Get into the tub, have a seat, and drop one bomb per bath.

NOTE: If you want your bath bombs to bubble, simply add ½ teaspoon of SLES powder (see page 11) to the dry mix. You can find a more detailed recipe on page 100.

2¼ CUPS (497 G) BAKING SODA

1¼ CUPS (288 G) GRANULAR CITRIC ACID

¼ CUP (24 G) CORNSTARCH

¾ CUP (180 ML) CANOLA, COCONUT, SWEET ALMOND (OUR FAVORITE), OR OTHER OIL

1 TEASPOON FRAGRANCE OR ESSENTIAL OIL

½+ TEASPOON LIQUID COLOR (ADD MORE OR LESS TO ACHIEVE YOUR DESIRED COLOR; SEE PAGE 10 FOR MORE DETAILS)

3–4 MOLDS

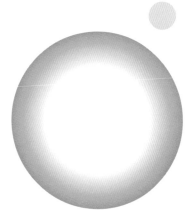

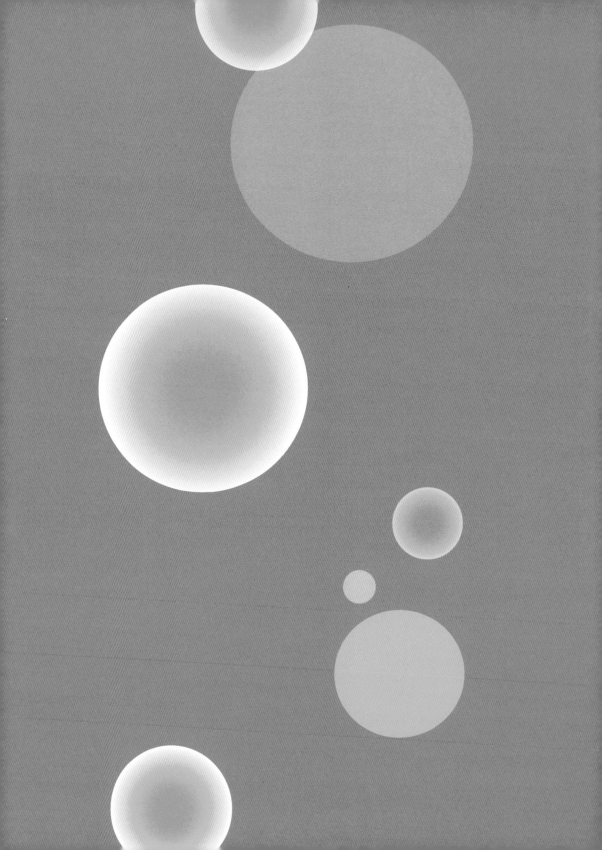

FRUITY FRAGRANCES

WHAT DO YOU GET WHEN YOU
COMBINE THE UNIQUE THRILL OF A
FIZZING BATH BOMB WITH THE TOTALLY
SATISFYING AROMA OF FRESH FRUIT?
COMPLETE BATH BLISS, OF COURSE!

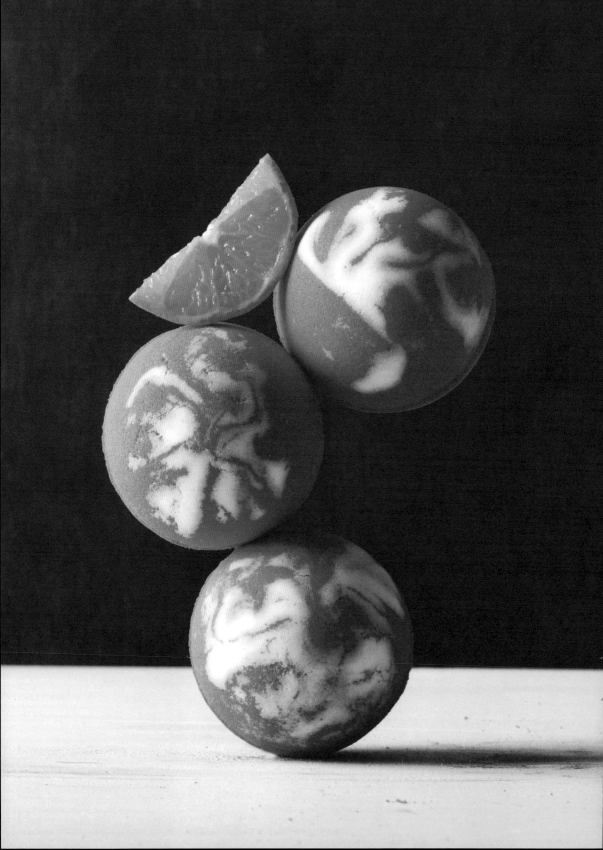

TANGERINE TEMPTER

WHO DOESN'T LOVE THE TANGY FRAGRANCE OF A FRESH, RIPE TANGERINE? THIS VIBRANT FIZZER WILL HAVE YOU CANCELING YOUR EVENING PLANS IN FAVOR OF A SOAK!

MAKES 3–4 BOMBS

1 In a large bowl, mix together the baking soda, citric acid, and cornstarch, and divide into two equal parts.

2 Separately, combine the oil and fragrance, and divide into two equal parts, coloring half orange and leave the other half uncolored.

3 Add the oil mixtures to each batch of dry ingredients and combine.

4 Mix each batch separately with your hands until each mixture becomes the consistency of wet sand. Wash and dry your hands between each mixing segment. (If you don't like to get your hands messy, you can wear rubber gloves for this part.) The more vigorous your mixing style, the better the ingredients will be distributed, so don't be shy. Five minutes of stirring, compressing, and kneading should do the trick.

5 As you press the mixture into the molds, gently swirl the orange and white mixes together with a spoon handle.

6 Press the mold halves together and let the bombs dry for 24–48 hours.

7 Once they are completely dry, remove them carefully from the molds. If you only have one mold, you can also gently remove the bombs as you make them and lay them out to dry on a flat surface. Try not to touch them until they harden.

2¼ CUPS (497 G) BAKING SODA

1¼ CUPS (288 G) GRANULAR CITRIC ACID

¼ CUP (24 G) CORNSTARCH

¾ CUP (180 ML) OIL

1 TEASPOON TANGERINE FRAGRANCE

½ TEASPOON ORANGE LIQUID COLOR

3–4 SPHERE-SHAPED MOLDS

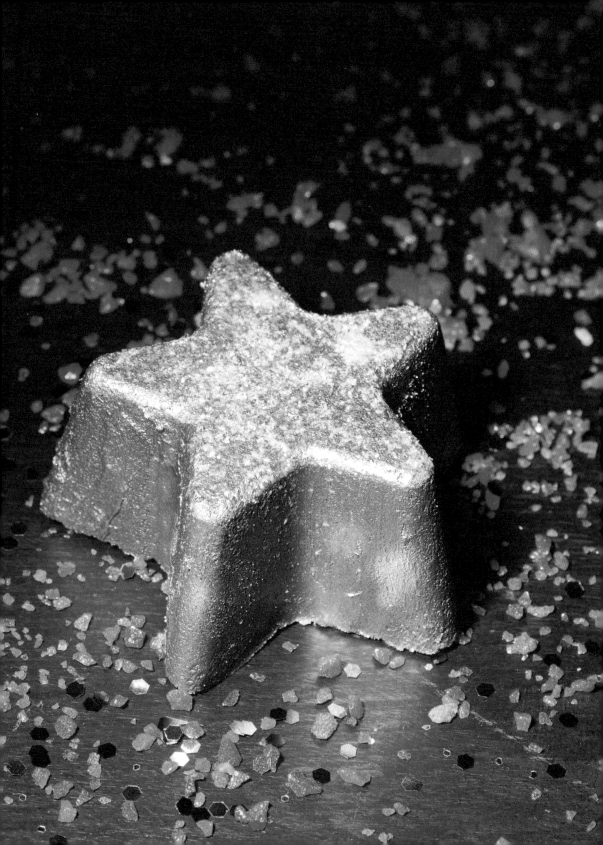

THIS ZESTY, LEMON-SCENTED BOMB HAS POPPING CANDY INSIDE FOR A FUN SURPRISE, MAKING IT A GREAT GIFT FOR THE SUPERSTAR IN YOUR LIFE. WARNING: MAY ATTRACT PAPARAZZI.

SUPER-STAR

MAKES 3–4 BOMBS

1 In a large bowl, mix together the baking soda, citric acid, and cornstarch.

2 In a separate bowl, combine the oil, fragrance, and liquid color.

3 Add the wet ingredients to the dry ingredients and mix with your hands until the mixture becomes the consistency of wet sand. (If you don't like to get your hands messy, you can wear rubber gloves for this part.) The more vigorous your mixing style, the better the ingredients will be distributed, so don't be shy. Five minutes of stirring, compressing, and kneading should do the trick.

4 Sprinkle the mix into a star-shaped mold, filling halfway.

5 Place 1 teaspoon of popping candy in the center of each bomb and top it off with more bath bomb mix, pressing firmly until the mold is filled completely.

6 Let stand until the bombs are hardened, 24–48 hours.

7 Once they are completely dry, remove them carefully from the molds. If you only have one mold, you can also gently remove the bombs as you make them and lay them out to dry on a flat surface. Try not to touch them until they harden.

8 Combine the mica with a few drops of rubbing alcohol and mix until a paste forms. Paint the mixture onto the surface of the bomb, covering it completely. Sprinkle eco glitter on top for a finishing touch.

2¼ CUPS (497 G) BAKING SODA

1¼ CUPS (288 G) GRANULAR CITRIC ACID

¼ CUP (24 G) CORNSTARCH

¾ CUP (180 ML) OIL

1 TEASPOON LEMON FRAGRANCE

½ TEASPOON YELLOW LIQUID COLOR

3–4 STAR-SHAPED MOLDS

1 TABLESPOON POPPING CANDY

1 TABLESPOON SILVER MICA POWDER

2 DROPS RUBBING ALCOHOL

½ TEASPOON ECO GLITTER

THE HEART-BREAKER

AS MUCH AS WE HATE TO ADMIT IT, LOVE DOESN'T ALWAYS LAST. ENTER THE HEARTBREAKER. THIS FRUITY FIZZER WILL LIFT YOUR SPIRITS AND HELP YOU GET YOUR MIND OFF YOUR WOES. (FOR THREE TO FIVE MINUTES, AT LEAST.)

MAKES
3–4
BOMBS

2¼ CUPS (497 G) BAKING SODA

1¼ CUPS (288 G) GRANULAR CITRIC ACID

¼ CUP (24 G) CORNSTARCH

¾ CUP (180 ML) OIL

1 TEASPOON GRAPE FRAGRANCE

¼ TEASPOON PINK LIQUID COLOR

¼ TEASPOON PURPLE LIQUID COLOR

3–4 HEART-SHAPED MOLDS

ALUMINUM FOIL

1 In a large bowl, mix together the baking soda, citric acid, and cornstarch, and divide into two equal parts.

2 Combine the oil and fragrance, and divide them into two equal parts, using the pink pigment to color the first part and the purple pigment to color the second part.

3 Add the oil mixtures to each batch of dry ingredients and combine.

4 Mix each batch separately with your hands until each mixture becomes the consistency of wet sand. Wash and dry your hands between each mixing segment. (If you don't like to get your hands messy, you can wear rubber gloves for this part.) The more vigorous your mixing style, the better the ingredients will be distributed, so don't be shy. Five minutes of stirring, compressing, and kneading should do the trick.

5 Create a divider down the center of the molds using a piece of aluminum foil folded lengthwise a few times and cut to size. This will create the broken heart effect. Then fill the mold and let the bombs dry for 24–48 hours.

6 Once they are completely dry, remove them carefully from the molds.

7 Next, imagine your crush ditching you. Now go ahead and cry a little bit. Yeah, girl. Let it all out. We feel you.

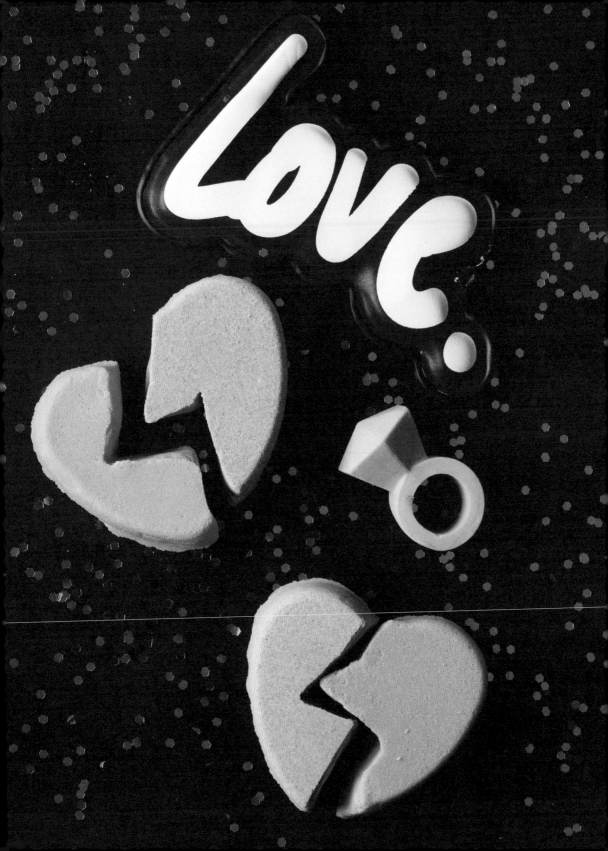

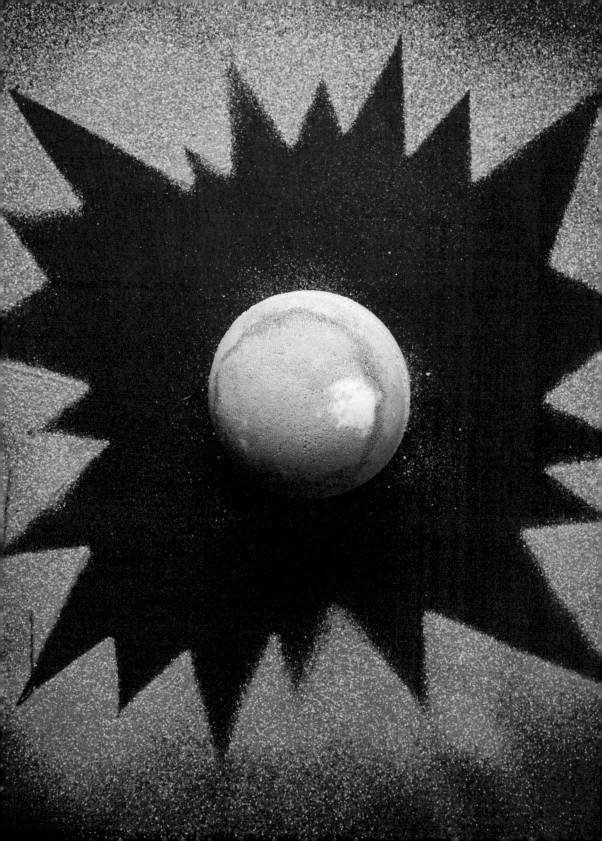

BLUEBERRY BLITZKRIEG

BEHOLD, THE POWER OF BLUEBERRY. WE SUPERCHARGED THIS EYE-POPPING FIZZER WITH A BOLD, JUICY FRAGRANCE AND TOPPED IT OFF WITH A VIBRANT MIX OF GORGEOUS COLORS. POW! TAKE THAT!

MAKES 3–4 BOMBS

1 In a large bowl, mix together the baking soda, citric acid, and cornstarch, and divide into two equal parts.

2 Next, take one of those parts and separate it into three more equal parts.

3 Separately, combine the oil and fragrance, and divide as above, coloring the largest part blue, and two of the smaller parts pink and purple. Leave the fourth part uncolored.

4 Add the oil mixtures to each batch of dry ingredients and combine.

5 Mix each batch separately with your hands until each mixture becomes the consistency of wet sand. Wash and dry your hands between each mixing segment. (If you don't like to get your hands messy, you can wear rubber gloves for this part.) The more vigorous your mixing style, the better the ingredients will be distributed, so don't be shy. Five minutes of stirring, compressing, and kneading should do the trick.

6 Add a pinch of pink, purple, and white mix to the molds. Sprinkle the perimeter generously with gold eco glitter.

7 Next, cover each half completely with the blue mix, press the mold halves together, and let the bombs dry for 24–48 hours.

8 Once they are completely dry, remove them carefully from the molds. If you only have one mold, you can also gently remove the bombs as you make them and lay them out to dry on a flat surface. Try not to touch them until they harden.

2¼ CUPS (497 G) BAKING SODA

1¼ CUPS (288 G) GRANULAR CITRIC ACID

¼ CUP (24 G) CORNSTARCH

¾ CUP (180 ML) OIL

1 TEASPOON BLUEBERRY FRAGRANCE

½ TEASPOON BLUE LIQUID COLOR

¼ TEASPOON PINK LIQUID COLOR

½ TEASPOON PURPLE LIQUID COLOR

3–4 SPHERE-SHAPED MOLDS

2 TEASPOONS GOLD ECO GLITTER

ZUMBA NIGHT

ISABEL WAS NOT LOOKING FORWARD TO HER SCHOOL ZUMBA UNIT—WHO WANTS TO LEARN TO DANCE IN FRONT OF RANDOM PEOPLE? BUT, MUCH TO HER SURPRISE, SHE BUSTED OUT SOME CRAZY ZUMBA MOVES AND ENDED UP LEADING THE CLASS! THIS BOMB IS PERFECT FOR ANYONE WHO NEEDS TO PSYCH THEMSELVES UP FOR A NEW CHALLENGE. (AND IF YOU AREN'T CURRENTLY CHALLENGING YOURSELF, MAYBE YOU SHOULD!)

MAKES 3–4 BOMBS

2¼ CUPS (497 G) BAKING SODA

1¼ CUPS (288 G) GRANULAR CITRIC ACID

¼ CUP (24 G) CORNSTARCH

¾ CUP (180 ML) OIL

1 TEASPOON STARFRUIT FRAGRANCE

¼ TEASPOON RED LIQUID COLOR

¼ TEASPOON YELLOW LIQUID COLOR

¼ TEASPOON ORANGE LIQUID COLOR

3–4 SPHERE-SHAPED MOLDS

1 In a large bowl, mix together the baking soda, citric acid, and cornstarch, and divide into three equal parts.

2 Separately, combine the oil and fragrance, and divide as above, coloring one part red, another part yellow, and the third part orange.

3 Add the oil mixtures to each batch of dry ingredients and combine.

4 Mix each batch separately with your hands until each mixture becomes the consistency of wet sand. Wash and dry your hands between each mixing segment. (If you don't like to get your hands messy, you can wear rubber gloves for this part.) The more vigorous your mixing style, the better the ingredients will be distributed, so don't be shy. Five minutes of stirring, compressing, and kneading should do the trick.

5 Use a half teaspoon to scoop the mix, layering all three colors into the molds. Overfill each half before combining. Press the mold halves together and let the bombs dry for 24–48 hours.

6 Once they are completely dry, remove them carefully from the molds. If you only have one mold, you can also gently remove the bombs as you make them and lay them out to dry on a flat surface. Try not to touch them until they harden.

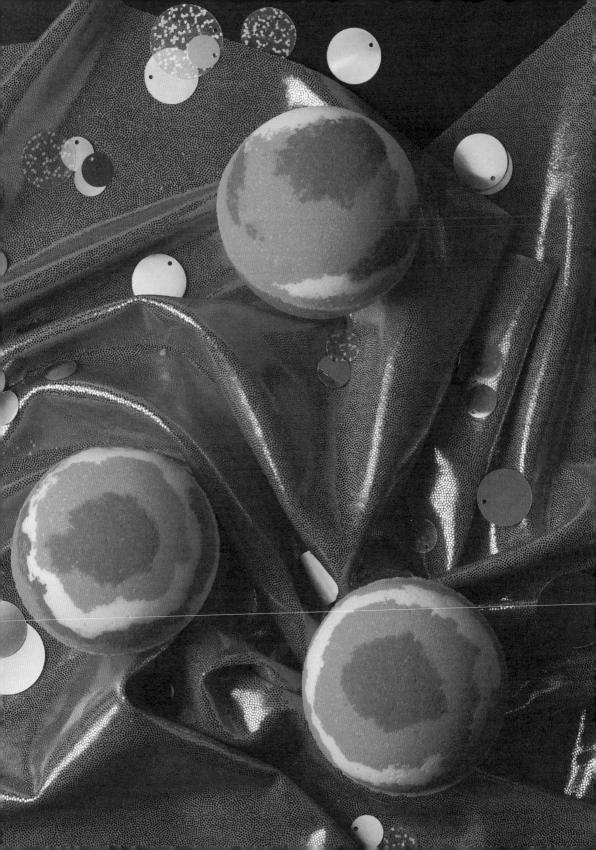

TIKI TIME

CREDIT HARRY FOR ANOTHER GREAT IDEA. (HE'S OUR YOUNGER BROTHER.) CREATOR OF THE NINJA BOMB, HERO BOMB, AND SPORTY BOMB THAT WE SELL IN STORES, HE ALSO NAMED THIS ONE FOR US.

MAKES 3-4 BOMBS

2¼ CUPS (497 G) BAKING SODA

1¼ CUPS (288 G) GRANULAR CITRIC ACID

¼ CUP (24 G) CORNSTARCH

¾ CUP (180 ML) OIL

1 TEASPOON BANANA FRAGRANCE

½ TEASPOON YELLOW LIQUID COLOR

3–4 TIKI HEAD–SHAPED MOLDS (FOUND ONLINE)

1   In a large bowl, mix together the baking soda, citric acid, and cornstarch.

2   In a separate bowl, combine the oil, fragrance, and liquid color.

3   Add the wet ingredients to the dry ingredients and mix with your hands until the mixture becomes the consistency of wet sand. (If you don't like to get your hands messy, you can wear rubber gloves for this part.) The more vigorous your mixing style, the better the ingredients will be distributed, so don't be shy. Five minutes of stirring, compressing, and kneading should do the trick.

4   Next, press the mixture firmly into the molds and let the bombs dry for 24–48 hours.

5   Once they are completely dry, remove them carefully from the molds. If you only have one mold, you can also gently remove the bombs as you make them and lay them out to dry on a flat surface. Try not to touch them until they harden.

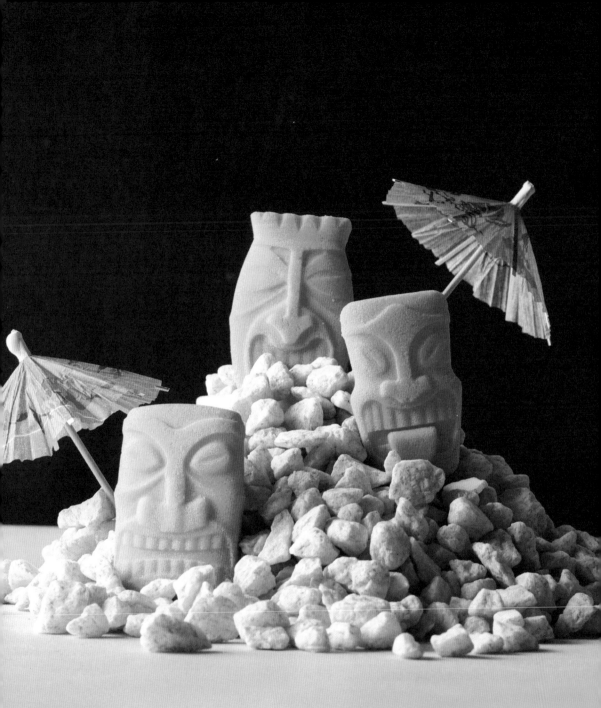

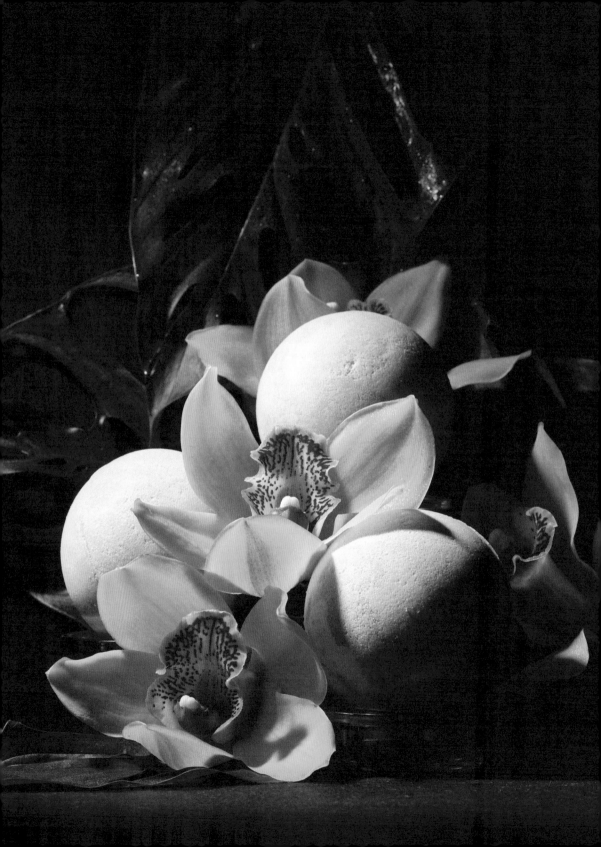

WE GOT TO VISIT SOME SOUTH PACIFIC ISLANDS RECENTLY, AND WERE AMAZED BY HOW FRAGRANT AND PERFECTLY RIPE THE FRUITS THERE WERE. WE ESPECIALLY LOVED THE GUAVA BECAUSE IT'S ONE OF THE LESSER APPRECIATED OF THE ISLAND FRUITS. WHY NOT BRING SOME OF THOSE FRESH, TROPICAL AROMAS INTO YOUR BATH? *AE KOA!* (THAT'S POLYNESIAN FOR "YES, PLEASE!")

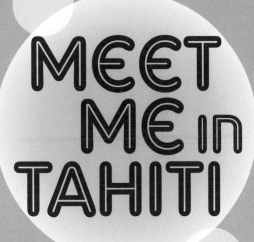

MEET ME IN TAHITI

MAKES
3–4
BOMBS

1 In a large bowl, mix together the baking soda, citric acid, and cornstarch, and divide into two equal parts.

2 Separately, combine the oil and fragrance, and divide into two equal parts, coloring half yellow and half blue.

3 Add the oil mixtures to each batch of dry ingredients and combine.

4 Mix each batch separately with your hands until each mixture becomes the consistency of wet sand. Wash and dry your hands between each mixing segment. (If you don't like to get your hands messy, you can wear rubber gloves for this part.) The more vigorous your mixing style, the better the ingredients will be distributed, so don't be shy. Five minutes of stirring, compressing, and kneading should do the trick.

5 Layer the colors in the molds and press the mold halves together. Then let the bombs dry for 24–48 hours.

6 Once they are completely dry, remove them carefully from the molds. If you only have one mold, you can also gently remove the bombs as you make them and lay them out to dry on a flat surface. Try not to touch them until they harden.

2¼ CUPS (497 G) BAKING SODA

1¼ CUPS (288 G) GRANULAR CITRIC ACID

¼ CUP (24 G) CORNSTARCH

¾ CUP (180 ML) OIL

1 TEASPOON GUAVA FRAGRANCE

¼ TEASPOON YELLOW LIQUID COLOR

¼ TEASPOON BLUE LIQUID COLOR

3–4 SPHERE-SHAPED MOLDS

CANDY CRUSH

SOMETIMES YOU HAVE A CRAVING FOR SOMETHING SWEET, BUT YOU DON'T WANT TO CHOW DOWN ON CANDY. ENTER THE CANDY CRUSH BATH BOMB. IT'LL HIT YOU WITH A BIG BLAST OF DECADENT FRAGRANCE THAT'LL GIVE YOU A WHOLE NEW KIND OF SUGAR RUSH!

MAKES 5-6 BOMBS

2¼ CUPS (497 G) BAKING SODA

1¼ CUPS (288 G) GRANULAR CITRIC ACID

¼ CUP (24 G) CORNSTARCH

¾ CUP (180 ML) OIL

¼ TEASPOON MARASCHINO CHERRY FRAGRANCE

¾ TEASPOON COTTON CANDY FRAGRANCE

½ TEASPOON PINK LIQUID COLOR

1 TEASPOON RAINBOW-COLORED CONFETTI SPRINKLES

5–6 CYLINDER-SHAPED MOLDS

1 In a large bowl, mix together the baking soda, citric acid, and cornstarch.

2 In a separate bowl, combine the oil, fragrances, and liquid color.

3 Add the wet ingredients to the dry ingredients and mix with your hands until the mixture becomes the consistency of wet sand. (If you don't like to get your hands messy, you can wear rubber gloves for this part.) The more vigorous your mixing style, the better the ingredients will be distributed, so don't be shy. Five minutes of stirring, compressing, and kneading should do the trick.

4 Sprinkle the rainbow-colored confetti sprinkles into the bottom of the mold before adding the bath bomb mix, pressing firmly so the topping adheres well to the bomb itself.

5 Next, press the mixture firmly into the molds and then let the bombs dry for 24–48 hours.

6 Once they are completely dry, remove them carefully from the mold. If you only have one mold, you can also gently remove the bombs as you make them and lay them out to dry on a flat surface. Try not to touch them until they harden.

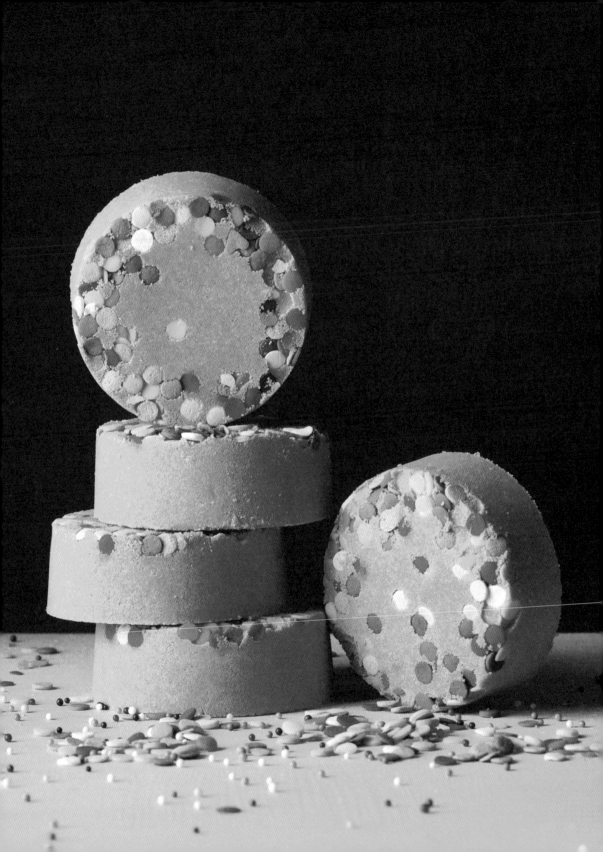

STRAWBERRY SUPERNOVA

WHEN YOU COMBINE
A POTENT KICK OF FRESH STRAWBERRIES WITH THE POWER OF THE COSMOS, THE RESULT IS OUT OF THIS WORLD!

MAKES
3–4
BOMBS

2¼ CUPS (497 G) BAKING SODA

1¼ CUPS (288 G) GRANULAR CITRIC ACID

¼ CUP (24 G) CORNSTARCH

¾ CUP (180 ML) OIL

1 TEASPOON STRAWBERRY FRAGRANCE

¼ TEASPOON RED LIQUID COLOR

¼ TEASPOON BLACK LIQUID COLOR

¼ TEASPOON PINK LIQUID COLOR

3–4 SPHERE-SHAPED MOLDS

1   In a large bowl, mix together the baking soda, citric acid, and cornstarch, and divide into two equal parts.

2   Next, take one of those parts and separate it into three more equal parts.

3   Separately, combine the oil and fragrance, and divide as above, coloring the largest part red, and two of the smaller parts black and pink. Leave the fourth part uncolored.

4   Add the oil mixtures to each batch of dry ingredients and combine.

5   Mix each batch separately with your hands until each mixture becomes the consistency of wet sand. Wash and dry your hands between each mixing segment. (If you don't like to get your hands messy, you can wear rubber gloves for this part.) The more vigorous your mixing style, the better the ingredients will be distributed, so don't be shy. Five minutes of stirring, compressing, and kneading should do the trick.

6   Add ½ teaspoon of pink, black, and white mix to each half of the mold.

7   Using a spoon handle, stir the mix to create a swirl effect.

8   Press the red mixture firmly into your molds, and then press the mold halves together. Let the bombs dry for 24–48 hours.

9   Once they are completely dry, remove them carefully from the molds. If you only have one mold, you can also gently remove the bombs as you make them and lay them out to dry on a flat surface. Try not to touch them until they harden.

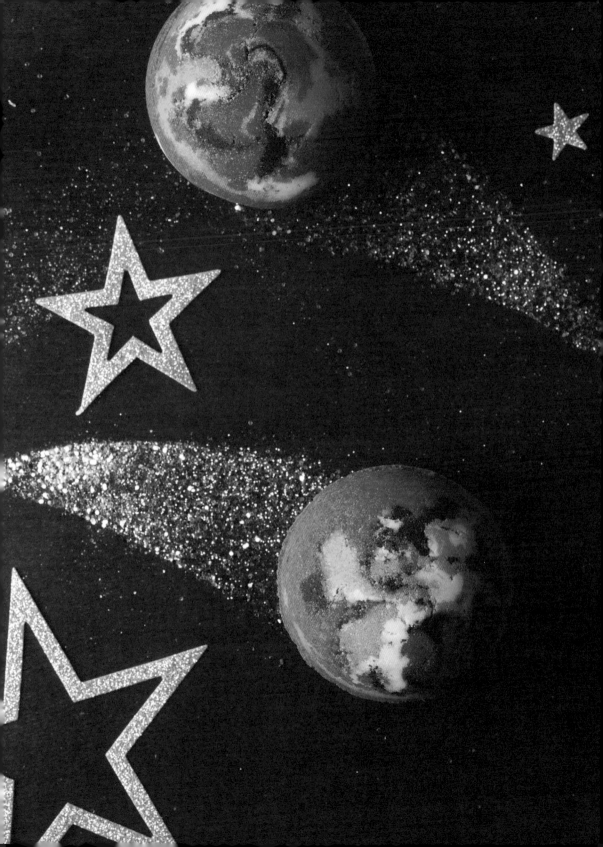

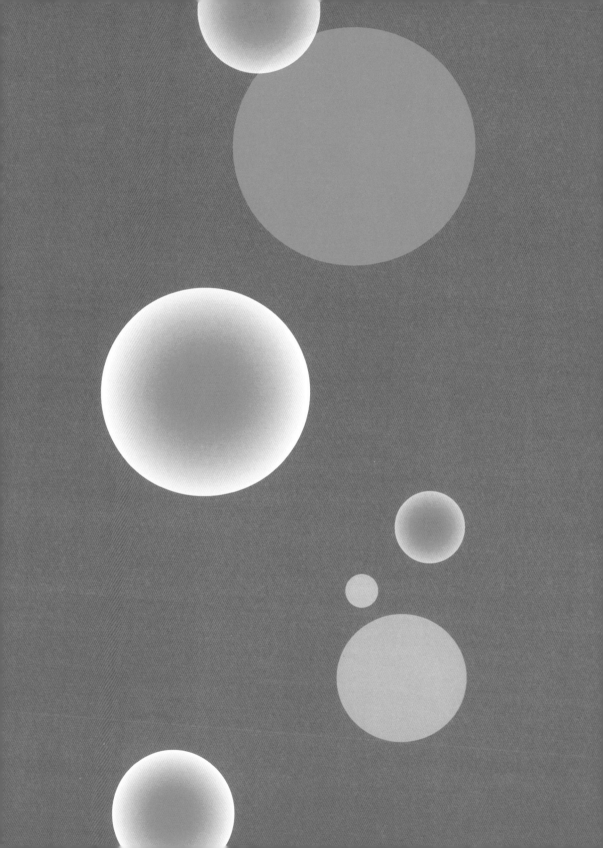

NUTTY + SPICY FRAGRANCES

IN A RUT? FEELING A BIT BLAND?
FIZZ YOURSELF OUT OF ANY FUNK
WHEN YOU EMBARK ON THIS EXCITING
FRAGRANCE ODYSSEY.

BRONZE GODDESS

THE AZTECS BELIEVED IN SUN GODS WHO BESTOWED LIGHT, WISDOM, AND LIFE ACROSS THE COSMOS. WHETHER YOU'RE LOOKING FOR SOME OF THAT OR JUST A RELAXING BATH, BRONZE GODDESS IS A GREAT CHOICE.

MAKES 3–4 BOMBS

2¼ CUPS (497 G) BAKING SODA

1¼ CUPS (288 G) GRANULAR CITRIC ACID

¼ CUP (24 G) CORNSTARCH

¾ CUP (180 ML) OIL

½ TEASPOON VANILLA FRAGRANCE

½ TEASPOON AMARETTO FRAGRANCE

3–4 SPHERE-SHAPED MOLDS

1 TABLESPOON COPPER-COLORED SPARKLE MICA POWDER

2–3 DROPS RUBBING ALCOHOL

1 In a large bowl, mix together the baking soda, citric acid, and cornstarch.

2 In a separate bowl, combine the oil and fragrances.

3 Add the wet ingredients to the dry ingredients and mix with your hands until the mixture becomes the consistency of wet sand. (If you don't like to get your hands messy, you can wear rubber gloves for this part.) The more vigorous your mixing style, the better the ingredients will be distributed, so don't be shy. Five minutes of stirring, compressing, and kneading should do the trick.

4 Next, press the mixture firmly into your molds, press the mold halves together, and then let the bombs dry for 24–48 hours.

5 Once they are completely dry, remove them carefully from the molds. If you only have one mold, you can also gently remove the bombs as you make them and lay them out to dry on a flat surface. Try not to touch them until they harden.

6 Use a paintbrush to mix a few drops of rubbing alcohol into the mica powder to form a paste and cover each bomb completely.

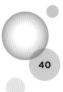

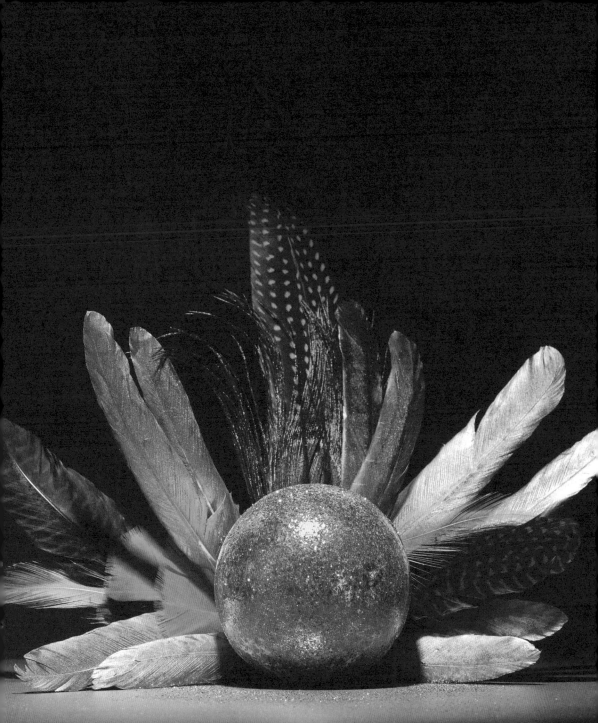

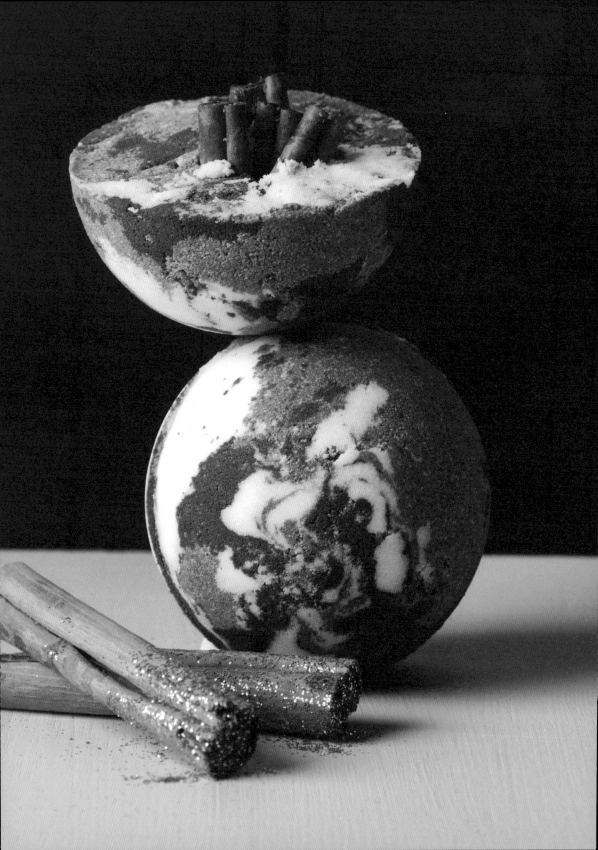

SOMETIMES A FRAGRANCE BRINGS YOU BACK TO YOUR CHILD-HOOD. THIS ONE REMINDS US OF WAKING UP ON A SUNDAY MORNING TO THE SWEET SMELL OF MADE-FROM-SCRATCH CINNAMON ROLLS BAKING IN THE OVEN. WHO DOESN'T LOVE THAT AROMA? THAT'S WHY WE CREATED CINNAMON TWIST. AND AS A BONUS, THERE ARE CINNAMON STICKS IN THE CENTER!

CINNAMON TWIST

MAKES
3–4
BOMBS

1 In a large bowl, mix together the baking soda, citric acid, and cornstarch, and divide into three equal parts.

2 Separately, combine the oil and fragrance, and divide as above.

3 In a small bowl, mix together the purple and yellow liquid colors to form a dark brown color.

4 Add enough of the color to the first part to create a dark brown hue, enough to give a light brown color to the second, and leave the third uncolored.

5 Add the oil mixtures to each batch of dry ingredients and combine.

6 Finally, in a large bowl, add all three batches together, but DO NOT mix.

7 Fill each mold, taking care to add a little bit of all three colors to each half of the mold to create a mixed-up effect.

8 Add cinnamon sticks to the center of one mold, and press the mold halves together. Let the bombs dry for 24–48 hours. At this point you'll probably feel hungry, so you might want to make some actual cinnamon rolls while waiting for these bombs to dry.

9 Once they are completely dry, remove them carefully from the molds. If you only have one mold, you can also gently remove the bombs as you make them and lay them out to dry on a flat surface. Try not to touch them until they harden.

2¼ CUPS (497 G) BAKING SODA

1¼ CUPS (288 G) GRANULAR CITRIC ACID

¼ CUP (24 G) CORNSTARCH

¾ CUP (180 ML) OIL

½ TEASPOON CINNAMON BUN FRAGRANCE

½ TEASPOON PURPLE LIQUID COLOR

2 TEASPOONS YELLOW LIQUID COLOR

3–4 SPHERE-SHAPED MOLDS

3 CINNAMON STICKS

BOYFRIEND BOMB

GUESS WHAT? GUYS LOVE BATH BOMBS, TOO! SO IF YOU WANT TO SURPRISE THE HANDSOME FELLA IN YOUR LIFE WITH A BATH TREAT OF HIS VERY OWN, THIS BOMB IS IT.

MAKES 3–4 BOMBS

2¼ CUPS (497 G) BAKING SODA

1¼ CUPS (288 G) GRANULAR CITRIC ACID

¼ CUP (24 G) CORNSTARCH

¾ CUP (180 ML) OIL

1 TEASPOON OAKMOSS FRAGRANCE

1 TEASPOON VETIVER FRAGRANCE

½ TEASPOON GREEN LIQUID COLOR

3–4 SPHERE-SHAPED MOLDS

1 In a large bowl, mix together the baking soda, citric acid, and cornstarch, and divide into two equal parts.

2 Combine the oil and fragrances, and divide them into two equal parts, using the green pigment to color the first part; leave the second part uncolored.

3 Add the oil mixtures to each batch of dry ingredients and combine.

4 Mix each batch separately with your hands until each mixture becomes the consistency of wet sand. Wash and dry your hands between each mixing segment. (If you don't like to get your hands messy, you can wear rubber gloves for this part.) The more vigorous your mixing style, the better the ingredients will be distributed, so don't be shy. Five minutes of stirring, compressing, and kneading should do the trick.

5 Using a ½ teaspoon, fill each mold with the mixes, one spoon at a time, alternating between green and white and pressing each layer flat to create a striped effect. For best results, overfill the molds before pressing the halves together. Let the bombs dry for 24–48 hours.

6 Once they are completely dry, remove them carefully from the molds. If you only have one mold, you can also gently remove the bombs as you make them and lay them out to dry on a flat surface. Try not to touch them until they harden.

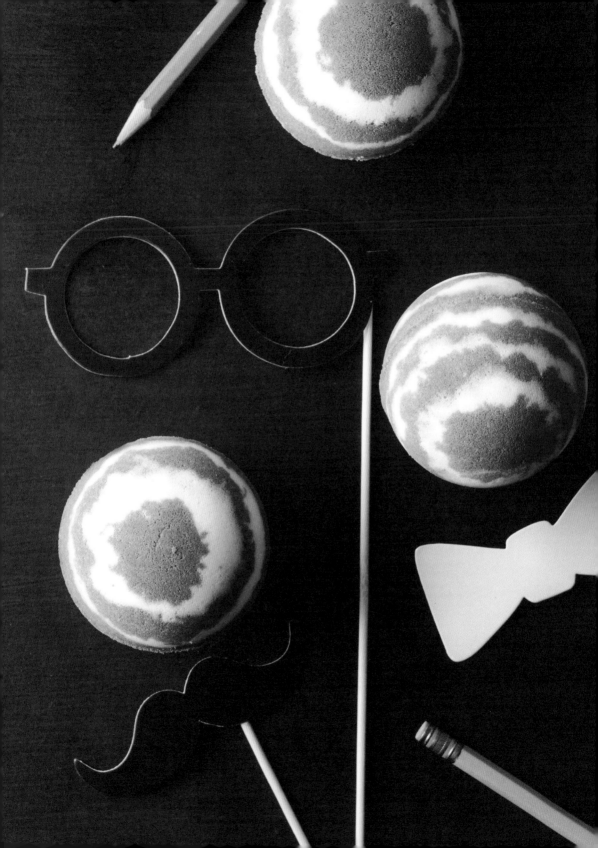

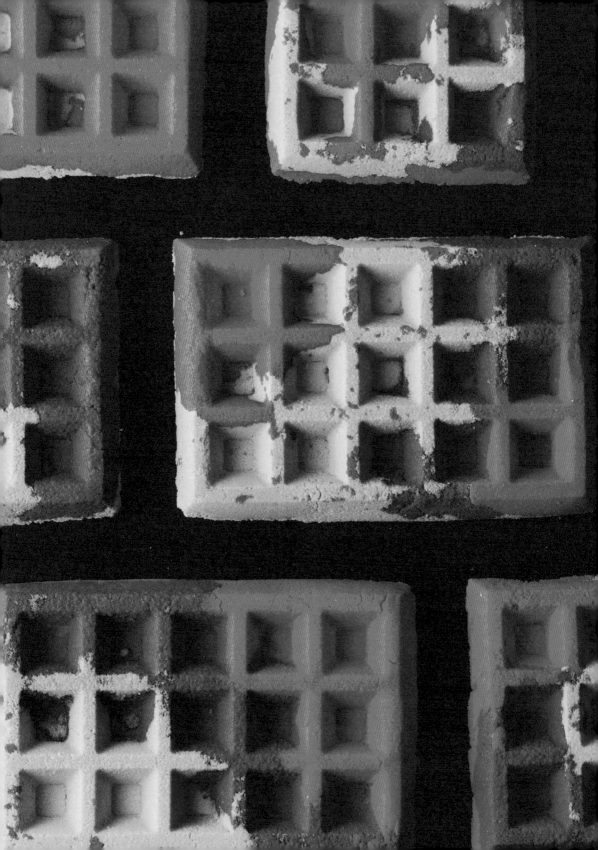

WAFFLE BOMB

NO ACTUAL BUTTER OR SYRUP REQUIRED. OUR WAFFLE BOMB IS A GREAT CHOICE IF YOU LIKE TO BATHE FIRST THING IN THE MORNING, AND IT'S A HECK OF A LOT PRETTIER THAN OUR OTHER IDEA, THE PANCAKE BOMB.

MAKES
3–4
BOMBS

1 In a large bowl, mix together the baking soda, citric acid, and cornstarch, and divide into three equal parts.

2 Separately, combine the oil and fragrance, and divide as above, coloring one part neon pink, another part neon green, and the third part neon purple.

3 Add the oil mixtures to each batch of dry ingredients and combine.

4 Mix each batch separately with your hands until each mixture becomes the consistency of wet sand. Wash and dry your hands between each mixing segment. (If you don't like to get your hands messy, you can wear rubber gloves for this part.) The more vigorous your mixing style, the better the ingredients will be distributed, so don't be shy. Five minutes of stirring, compressing, and kneading should do the trick.

5 Next, press the mixture firmly into your molds and then let the bombs dry for 24–48 hours.

6 Once they are completely dry, remove them carefully from the molds. If you only have one mold, you can also gently remove the bombs as you make them and lay them out to dry on a flat surface. Try not to touch them until they harden.

2¼ CUPS (497 G) BAKING SODA

1¼ CUPS (288 G) GRANULAR CITRIC ACID

¼ CUP (24 G) CORNSTARCH

¾ CUP (180 ML) OIL

1 TEASPOON MAPLE SYRUP FRAGRANCE

¼ TEASPOON NEON PINK LIQUID COLOR

¼ TEASPOON NEON GREEN LIQUID COLOR

¼ TEASPOON NEON PURPLE LIQUID COLOR

3–4 WAFFLE-SHAPED MOLDS

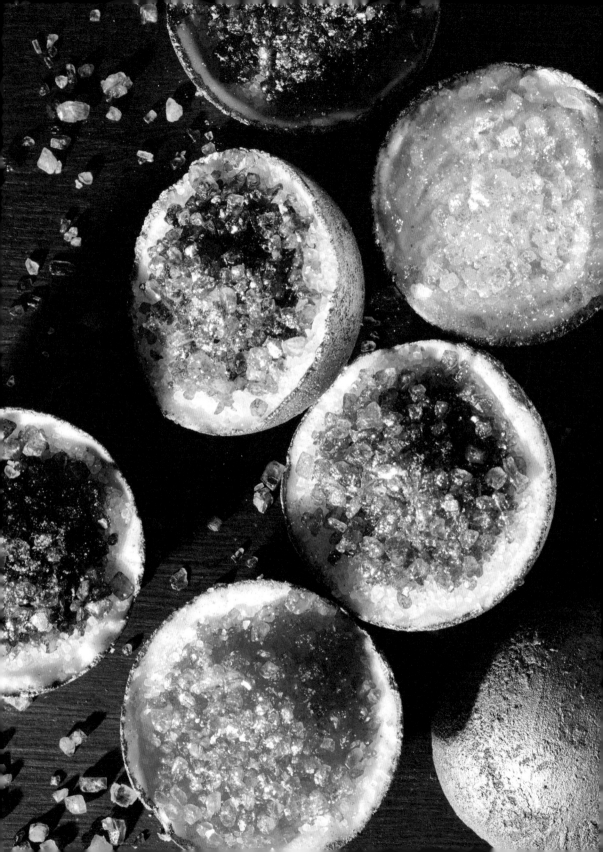

GEODES ARE SPARKLY
ROCK FORMATIONS THAT COME
FROM DEEP WITHIN THE EARTH,
WHERE THEY FORM SLOWLY
OVER THOUSANDS OF YEARS.
THANKFULLY, THESE LITTLE
BEAUTIES DON'T TAKE QUITE AS
LONG TO MAKE AND THEY SMELL
AS GOOD AS THEY LOOK.

GEODE BOMB

MAKES
3–4
BOMBS

1 In a large bowl, mix together the baking soda, citric acid, and cornstarch.

2 In a separate bowl, combine the oil and fragrance.

3 Add the wet ingredients to the dry ingredients and mix with your hands until the mixture becomes the consistency of wet sand. (If you don't like to get your hands messy, you can wear rubber gloves for this part.) The more vigorous your mixing style, the better the ingredients will be distributed, so don't be shy. Five minutes of stirring, compressing, and kneading should do the trick.

4 Press a ½-inch (13 mm) layer of bath bomb mix into the mold. The sides should be higher than the center, like the peel of a hollowed-out orange, and the edges should be a bit ragged. Allow to dry completely before removing from the molds.

5 Next, add a few drops of rubbing alcohol to the silver mica. Stir until a thin paste forms. With a paintbrush, paint the outside of the bomb with the paste. Let sit for 1 hour.

6 Add approximately 1 tablespoon of coarse sea salt to each painted half sphere, making sure to spread the salt to the outer edges of the half sphere.

7 Next, add 12–15 drops of liquid color to the 8 remaining tablespoons of coarse sea salt and mix well to distribute the color.

8 Add the colored sea salt to the center of the bomb and spread it out, as desired. Note: Spreading it to the very outer edge of the mold will create the most realistic-looking geode.

9 Heat the coconut oil in the microwave for a few seconds to melt it. Using a pipette or spoon, distribute the coconut oil, drop by drop, over the sea salt to bind it together.

10 Let harden and sprinkle the eco glitter on top to complete the look.

2¼ CUPS (497 G) BAKING SODA

1¼ CUPS (288 G) GRANULAR
CITRIC ACID

¼ CUP (24 G) CORNSTARCH

¾ CUP (180 ML) OIL

1 TEASPOON CANYON SPICE FRAGRANCE

3–4 HALF-SPHERE MOLDS

2–3 DROPS RUBBING ALCOHOL

1 TABLESPOON SILVER MICA

12 TABLESPOONS OF COARSE SEA SALT

12–15 DROPS LIQUID COLOR
OF YOUR CHOICE

1 TEASPOON COCONUT OIL

½ TEASPOON ECO GLITTER

FLORAL FRAGRANCES

GIVE YOURSELF A HEALTHY BURST
OF SPRING ANY TIME OF THE YEAR
WHEN YOU TREAT YOURSELF
TO THESE BATH BOMBS WITH
GORGEOUS FLORAL AROMAS.

FLOWER POWER

MAKES 3–4 BOMBS

WE'VE ALL SEEN BATH BOMBS WITH DRIED FLOWER PETALS ON TOP. THIS BOLD, BLACK UPDATE REPLACES THE TYPICAL POTPOURRI CREATION WITH SOMETHING A BIT MORE UNEXPECTED. IT'S PURE FLOWER POWER, COMPLEMENTED BY THE INTENSE, FLORAL PUNCH OF MAGNOLIA BLOSSOM—AND, FOR A FINISHING TOUCH, GOLD LEAF!

2¼ CUPS (497 G) BAKING SODA

1¼ CUPS (288 G) GRANULAR CITRIC ACID

¼ CUP (24 G) CORNSTARCH

¾ CUP (180 ML) OIL

1 TEASPOON MAGNOLIA BLOSSOM FRAGRANCE

3 TEASPOONS BLACK LIQUID COLOR

4 TEASPOONS DRIED FLOWER PETALS*

SQUARE-SHAPED MOLDS

1 TEASPOON GOLD LEAF

1 In a large bowl, mix together the baking soda, citric acid, and cornstarch.

2 In a separate bowl, combine the oil, fragrance, and liquid color.

3 Add the wet ingredients to the dry ingredients and mix with your hands until the mixture becomes the consistency of wet sand. (If you don't like to get your hands messy, you can wear rubber gloves for this part.) The more vigorous your mixing style, the better the ingredients will be distributed, so don't be shy. Five minutes of stirring, compressing, and kneading should do the trick.

4 Carefully lay the flower petals and gold leaf into the bottom and sides of the empty molds.

5 Next, press the mixture firmly into the molds, and then let the bombs dry for 24–48 hours.

6 Once they are completely dry, remove them carefully from the molds. If you only have one mold, you can also gently remove the bombs as you make them and lay them out to dry on a flat surface. Try not to touch them until they harden.

* Instead of breaking the budget on store-bought flower petals, pick some fresh ones from your yard or garden. For best results, pick them at their peak and speed up the drying process by placing them between two paper towels sandwiched between two microwave-safe plates; heat for 1 minute on high power. Uncover and let stand for a few days until completely dry, or the moisture in the petals could set off a fizzing reaction in your bath bombs.

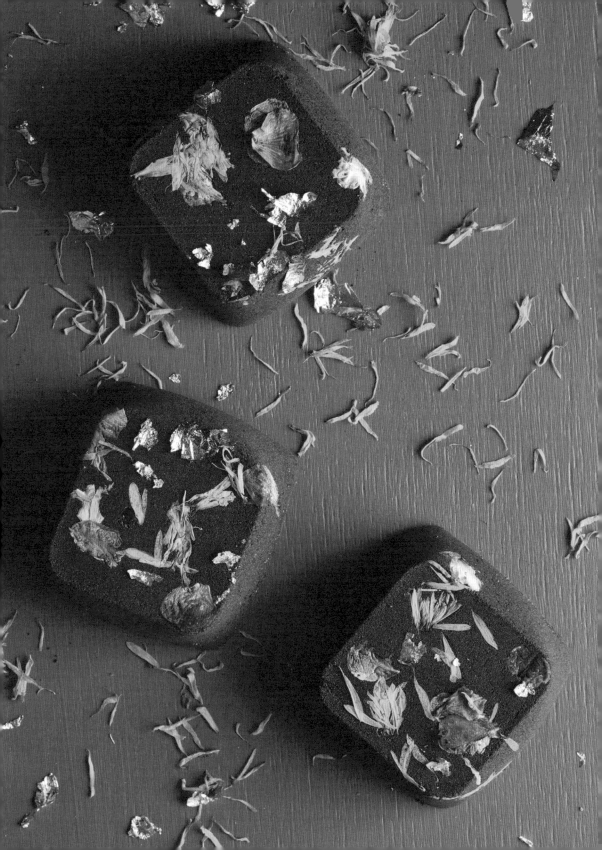

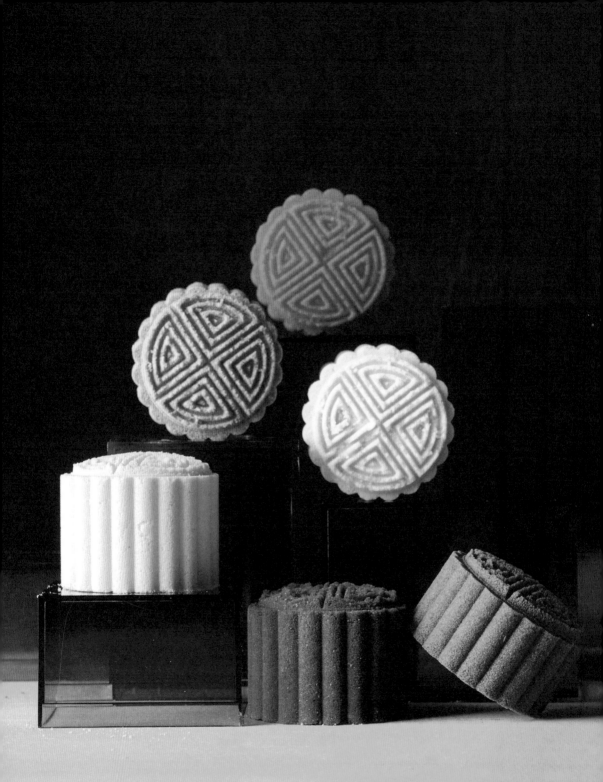

SOMEONE THINKS YOU'RE HOT. YOU'VE BEEN VOTED MOST LIKELY TO SURVIVE A ZOMBIE APOCALYPSE. WHATEVER MESSAGE YOU'RE TRYING TO CONVEY, THERE'S SOMETHING INCREDIBLY EXCITING ABOUT SENDING (AND RECEIVING!) A SECRET MESSAGE. YOU PICK THE PERSON, YOU PICK THE MESSAGE. NOW ALL YOU HAVE TO DO IS GET THE PERSON NEAR A TUB.

SECRET MESSAGE BOMB

MAKES 5–6 BOMBS

1 In a large bowl, mix together the baking soda, citric acid, and cornstarch.

2 In a separate bowl, combine the oil, fragrance, and liquid color.

3 Add the wet ingredients to the dry ingredients and mix with your hands until the mixture becomes the consistency of wet sand. (If you don't like to get your hands messy, you can wear rubber gloves for this part.) The more vigorous your mixing style, the better the ingredients will be distributed, so don't be shy. Five minutes of stirring, compressing, and kneading should do the trick.

4 Next, press some of the mixture loosely into the molds, filling it halfway.

5 Fold the secret messages into thirds and place one into the center of each partially filled mold. Add the remaining mix, press firmly, and let the bombs dry for 24–48 hours.

6 Once they are completely dry, remove them carefully from the molds. If you only have one mold, you can also gently remove the bombs as you make them and lay them out to dry on a flat surface. Try not to touch them until they harden.

* To make the messages, handwrite each message in pencil or permanent ink on a small piece of paper roughly the size of a fortune cookie message. You can also print the messages on a home laser printer. For extra durability, you can laminate the message or use waterproof paper, which can be purchased online.

2¼ CUPS (497 G) BAKING SODA

1¼ CUPS (288 G) GRANULAR CITRIC ACID

¼ CUP (24 G) CORNSTARCH

¾ CUP (180 ML) OIL

1 TEASPOON HONEYSUCKLE FRAGRANCE

½ TEASPOON LIQUID COLOR OF YOUR CHOICE

5–6 RUBBER MOLDS

SECRET MESSAGES*

YEAH, BABY!
GENDER-REVEAL BOMBS

MAKES 3–4 BOMBS

THROWING A BABY SHOWER FOR YOUR FAVORITE AUNT? THIS FIZZER MAKES A FUN, CLEVER SHOWER FAVOR THAT WILL ADD EXCITEMENT TO ANY GATHERING. (DON'T BE SURPRISED IF GUESTS SNEAK OFF TO THE NEAREST TUB OR SINK TO GET THE BABY GENDER SCOOP.)

2¼ CUPS (497 G) BAKING SODA

1¼ CUPS (288 G) GRANULAR CITRIC ACID

¼ CUP (24 G) CORNSTARCH

¾ CUP (180 ML) OIL

1 TEASPOON BABY'S BREATH FRAGRANCE

¼ TEASPOON PINK LIQUID COLOR

¼ TEASPOON BLUE LIQUID COLOR

3–4 SPHERE-SHAPED MOLDS

BABY GENDER MESSAGES*

1 In a large bowl, mix together the baking soda, citric acid, and cornstarch, and divide into two equal parts.

2 Separately, combine the oil and fragrance, and divide into two equal parts, coloring half pink and half blue.

3 Add the oil mixtures to each batch of dry ingredients and combine.

4 Mix each batch separately with your hands until each mixture becomes the consistency of wet sand. Wash and dry your hands between each mixing segment. (If you don't like to get your hands messy, you can wear rubber gloves for this part.) The more vigorous your mixing style, the better the ingredients will be distributed, so don't be shy. Five minutes of stirring, compressing, and kneading should do the trick.

5 Overfill half of the molds with pink mix and the other half with the blue.

6 Fold the secret messages into thirds and place one into the center of each pink mold. Press firmly, press the mold halves together firmly, and let the bombs dry for 24–48 hours.

7 Once they are completely dry, remove them carefully from the molds. If you only have one mold, you can also gently remove the bombs as you make them and lay them out to dry on a flat surface. Try not to touch them until they harden.

* To make the messages, handwrite each message in pencil or permanent ink on a small piece of paper roughly the size of a fortune cookie message. You can also print the messages on a home laser printer. For extra durability, you can laminate the message or use waterproof paper, which can be purchased online.

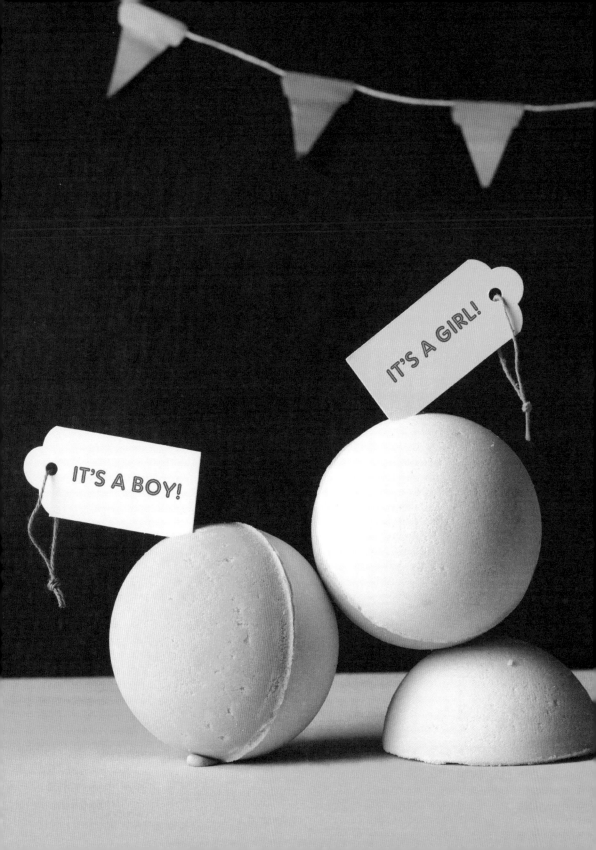

PROM-POSAL

MAKES 3–4 BOMBS

ASKING SOMEONE TO PROM OFTEN INVOLVES GRAND GESTURES, TIME, AND EFFORT. IF HIRING AN AIRPLANE TO WRITE YOUR PROM-POSAL IN THE SKY ISN'T A REALISTIC OPTION, HOW ABOUT POPPING THE QUESTION VIA A MESSAGE IN THE CENTER OF A FIZZING BATH BOMB?

2¼ CUPS (497 G) BAKING SODA

1¼ CUPS (288 G) GRANULAR CITRIC ACID

¼ CUP (24 G) CORNSTARCH

¾ CUP (180 ML) OIL

1 TEASPOON VERBENA FRAGRANCE

4 TEASPOONS PEARLESCENT CANDY TOPPING

3–4 SPHERE-SHAPED MOLDS

PROM-POSAL MESSAGES*

1 In a large bowl, mix together the baking soda, citric acid, and cornstarch.

2 In a separate bowl, combine the oil and fragrance.

3 Add the wet ingredients to the dry ingredients and mix with your hands until the mixture becomes the consistency of wet sand. (If you don't like to get your hands messy, you can wear rubber gloves for this part.) The more vigorous your mixing style, the better the ingredients will be distributed, so don't be shy. Five minutes of stirring, compressing, and kneading should do the trick.

4 Pour 1 teaspoon of pearlescent candy topping into the top half of the mold, loosely add the bath bomb mix, press the prom-posal message into the center, and add more mix.

5 Fill the bottom half with mix. Press the mold halves together and then let the bombs dry for 24–48 hours.

6 Once they are completely dry, remove them carefully from the molds. If you only have one mold, you can also gently remove the bombs as you make them and lay them out to dry on a flat surface. Try not to touch them until they harden.

* To make the messages, handwrite each message in pencil or permanent ink on a small piece of paper roughly the size of a fortune cookie message. You can also print the messages on a home laser printer. For extra durability, you can laminate the message or use waterproof paper, which can be purchased online.

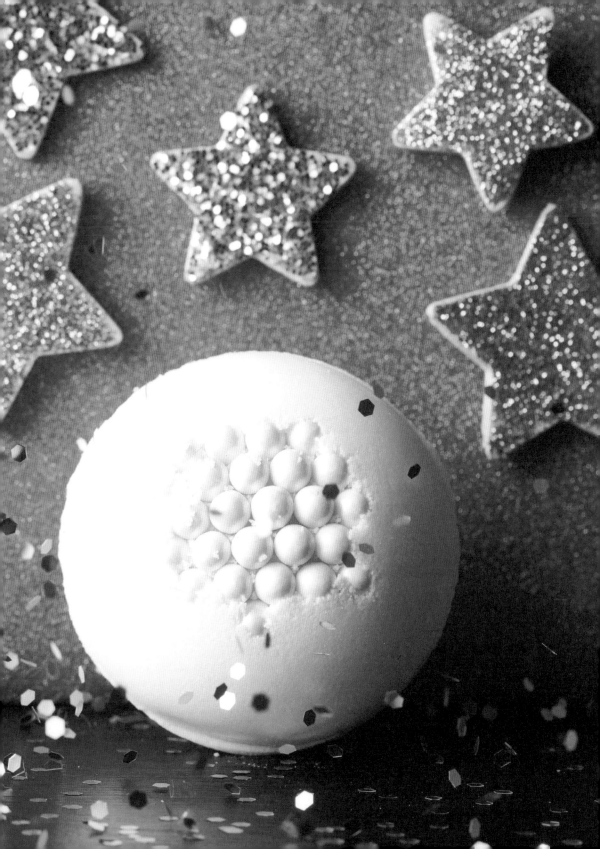

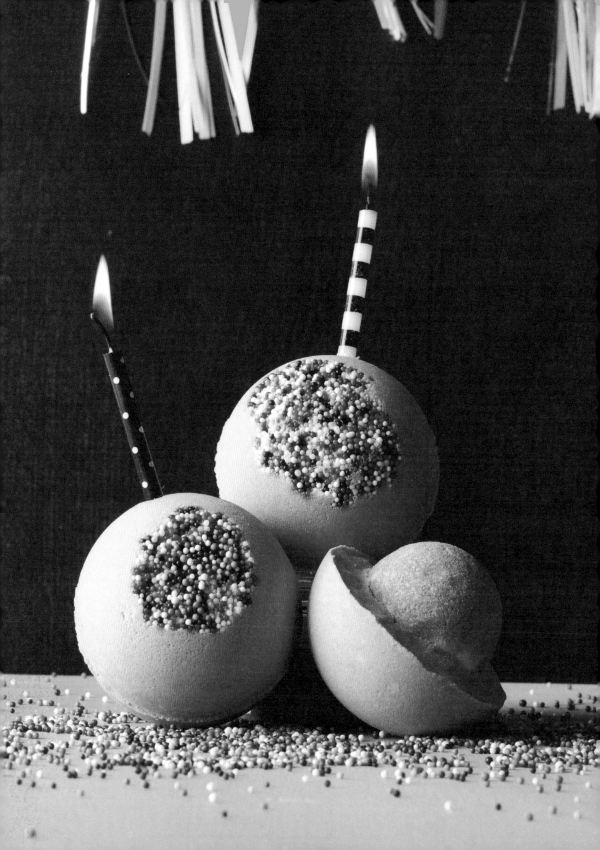

THIS CAKE-SCENTED

BOMB IS SO SPECIAL YOU'LL FEEL LIKE IT'S YOUR BIRTHDAY EVERY TIME YOU USE IT. AND WHEN THE OUTSIDE FIZZES AWAY, YOU'LL RECEIVE A GIFT IN THE FORM OF A FRAGRANT, DEEP PURPLE CORE.

NOTE: THIS RECIPE SHOULD BE MADE IN TWO STAGES, OVER TWO DAYS.

COLOR-CHANGING
BIRTHDAY
BOMB

MAKES 3–4 BOMBS

1 In a large bowl, mix together the baking soda, citric acid, and cornstarch. Separate the mix into two halves.

2 In a smaller bowl, combine half of the oil, the amaretto fragrance, and the purple color.

3 Add the wet ingredients to the dry ingredients and mix each batch separately with your hands until each mixture becomes the consistency of wet sand. Wash and dry your hands between each mixing segment. (If you don't like to get your hands messy, you can wear rubber gloves for this part.) The more vigorous your mixing style, the better the ingredients will be distributed, so don't be shy. Five minutes of stirring, compressing, and kneading should do the trick.

4 Press the bomb mixture into the 1¾-inch (4.5 cm) sphere-shaped molds, press the halves together, and let them dry for 24–48 hours before moving to the next step. Carefully remove them from the molds.

5 To make the outer bomb, combine the remaing half of the oil, the cake fragrance, and the magenta color. Mix the wet and remaining dry ingredients.

6 Sprinkle 1 teaspoon of the rainbow nonpareils and 1 heaping teaspoon of magenta mix into the top of each 2¾-inch (7 cm) mold. Carefully place one 1¾-inch (4.5 cm) purple bomb into the mold. Pack the magenta mix around the smaller bomb and cover it completely, overfilling the mold. Do your best to place the smaller bomb in the middle of the larger bomb.

7 Fill the bottom of the mold with magenta mix. Press the halves together, and then let the bombs dry for 24–48 hours.

8 Once they are completely dry, remove them carefully from the molds. If you only have one mold, you can also gently remove the bombs as you make them and lay them out to dry on a flat surface. Try not to touch them until they harden.

2¼ CUPS (497 G) BAKING SODA

1¼ CUPS (288 G) GRANULAR CITRIC ACID

¼ CUP (24 G) CORNSTARCH

¾ CUP (180 ML) OIL

½ TEASPOON AMARETTO FRAGRANCE

½ TEASPOON PURPLE LIQUID COLOR

3–4 1¾-INCH (4.5 CM) SPHERE-SHAPED MOLDS (FOR THE INNER BOMBS)

½ TEASPOON CAKE FRAGRANCE

¼ TEASPOON MAGENTA LIQUID COLOR

2 TABLESPOONS RAINBOW NONPAREILS

3–4 2¾-INCH (7 CM) SPHERE-SHAPED MOLDS (FOR THE OUTER BOMBS)

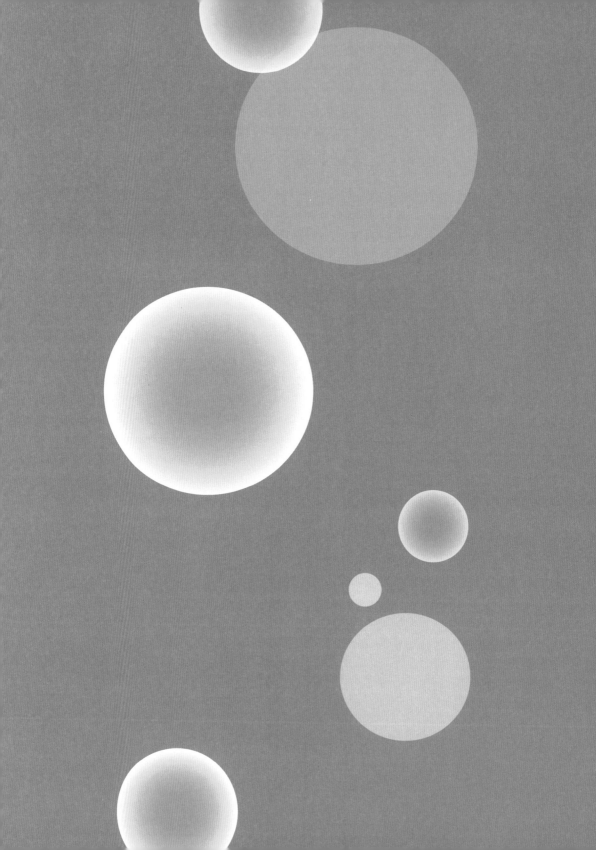

AROMATHERAPY FRAGRANCES

SOMETIMES A MERE FRAGRANCE ISN'T ENOUGH TO MAKE YOU FEEL YOUR BEST. SOMETIMES YOU NEED THERAPY. THAT'S RIGHT: AROMATHERAPY. WHETHER YOU'RE SEEKING RELAXATION, A BOOST OF ENERGY, OR RELIEF FROM A STUBBORN COLD, THE FIZZERS THAT FOLLOW CONTAIN THE VALUE-ADDED KICK OF FRAGRANCES THAT ARE KNOWN TO OFFER TANGIBLE HEALTH BENEFITS WHEN INHALED.

STRESS CASE

MONDAYS. TRAFFIC. HOMEWORK. CHORES. WHATEVER YOUR TRIGGERS ARE, WHEN YOU FEEL LIKE A BALL OF STRESS, SIMPLY DROP THIS BOMB, TAKE A FEW DEEP BREATHS, AND . . . *VOILÀ!* CASE CLOSED.

MAKES
3–4
BOMBS

2¼ CUPS (497 G) BAKING SODA

1¼ CUPS (288 G) GRANULAR CITRIC ACID

¼ CUP (24 G) CORNSTARCH

¾ CUP (180 ML) OIL

1 TEASPOON LAVENDER FRAGRANCE

½ TEASPOON GREEN LIQUID COLOR

¼ TEASPOON YELLOW LIQUID COLOR

¼ TEASPOON PURPLE LIQUID COLOR

3–4 SPHERE-SHAPED MOLDS

1 Mix together the baking soda, citric acid, and cornstarch, and divide into two equal parts.

2 Next, take one half and separate it in half again.

3 Separately, combine the oil and fragrance, and divide as above, coloring the largest part green, and the two smaller parts yellow and purple.

4 Add the oil mixtures to each batch of dry ingredients and combine.

5 Mix each batch separately with your hands until each mixture becomes the consistency of wet sand. Wash and dry your hands between each mixing segment. (If you don't like to get your hands messy, you can wear rubber gloves for this part.) The more vigorous your mixing style, the better the ingredients will be distributed, so don't be shy. Five minutes of stirring, compressing, and kneading should do the trick.

6 Spoon 1 teaspoon of purple, green, and yellow into each half of the mold, swirl with a spoon handle, and add green mix to fill up the mold and press the mixture firmly into your molds. Press the mold halves together and then let the bombs dry for 24–48 hours.

7 Once they are completely dry, remove them carefully from the molds. If you only have one mold, you can also gently remove the bombs as you make them and lay them out to dry on a flat surface. Try not to touch them until they harden.

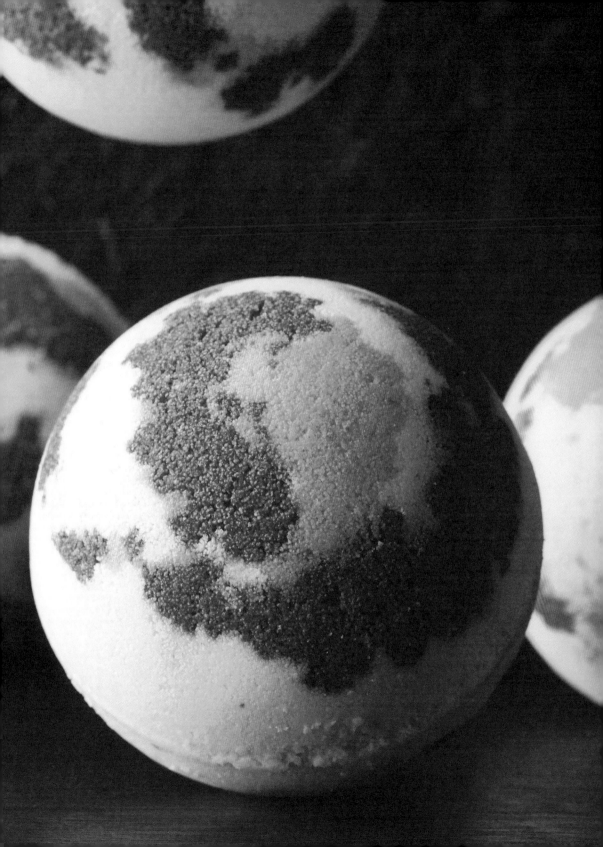

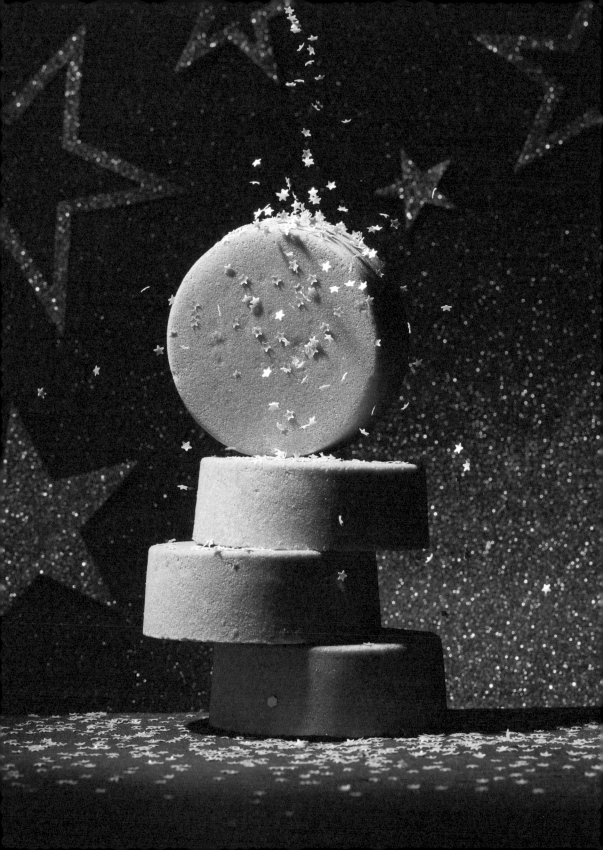

THE WORST KIND OF ALL-NIGHTER IS THE ONE YOU NEVER INTENDED ON PULLING. SO PREPARE IN ADVANCE FOR A SOLID BLOCK OF SHUT-EYE WITH THIS RELAXING, FLORAL-SCENTED BATH BOMB.

THE INSOMNIAC

MAKES 5–6 BOMBS

1 In a large bowl, mix together the baking soda, citric acid, and cornstarch.

2 In a separate bowl, combine the oil, fragrance, and liquid color.

3 Add the wet ingredients to the dry ingredients and mix with your hands until the mixture becomes the consistency of wet sand. (If you don't like to get your hands messy, you can wear rubber gloves for this part.) The more vigorous your mixing style, the better the ingredients will be distributed, so don't be shy. Five minutes of stirring, compressing, and kneading should do the trick.

4 Next, press the mixture firmly into your molds and then let the bombs dry for 24–48 hours.

5 Once they are completely dry, remove them carefully from the molds. If you only have one mold, you can also gently remove the bombs as you make them and lay them out to dry on a flat surface. Try not to touch them until they harden.

6 Finally, sprinkle stars liberally over the bombs.

2¼ CUPS (497 G) BAKING SODA

1¼ CUPS (288 G) GRANULAR CITRIC ACID

¼ CUP (24 G) CORNSTARCH

¾ CUP (180 ML) OIL

1 TEASPOON JASMINE FRAGRANCE

1 TEASPOON BLUE LIQUID COLOR

5–6 CYLINDER-SHAPED MOLDS

3 TEASPOONS EDIBLE SILVER METALLIC STARS

LESS PAIN, MORE GAIN

MAKES 3–4 BOMBS

WHEN WE FIRST DECIDED TO TRY MAKING BATH BOMBS, IT WAS BECAUSE OUR MUSCLES HURT FROM SPORTS AND WE WANTED RELIEF! THESE BOMBS CONTAIN PEPPERMINT AND SEA SALTS, WHICH ARE GREAT FOR SORE MUSCLES.

2¼ CUPS (497 G) BAKING SODA

1¼ CUPS (288 G) GRANULAR CITRIC ACID

¼ CUP (24 G) CORNSTARCH

¾ CUP (180 ML) OIL

1 TEASPOON PEPPERMINT FRAGRANCE

½ TEASPOON PURPLE LIQUID COLOR

4 TEASPOONS COARSE BLACK SEA SALT

3–4 SPHERE-SHAPED MOLDS

1 In a large bowl, mix together the baking soda, citric acid, and cornstarch.

2 In a separate bowl, combine the oil, fragrance, and liquid color.

3 Add the wet ingredients to the dry ingredients and mix with your hands until the mixture becomes the consistency of wet sand. (If you don't like to get your hands messy, you can wear rubber gloves for this part.) The more vigorous your mixing style, the better the ingredients will be distributed, so don't be shy. Five minutes of stirring, compressing, and kneading should do the trick.

4 Mix in the black sea salt to the mixture.

5 Next, press the mixture firmly into your molds, press the mold halves together, and then let the bombs dry for 24–48 hours.

6 Once they are completely dry, remove them carefully from the molds. If you only have one mold, you can also gently remove the bombs as you make them and lay them out to dry on a flat surface. Try not to touch them until they harden.

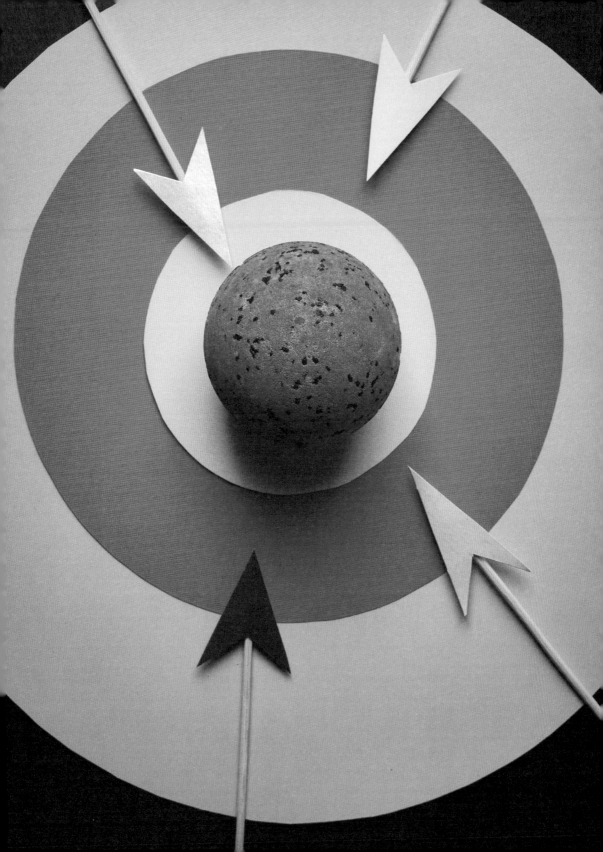

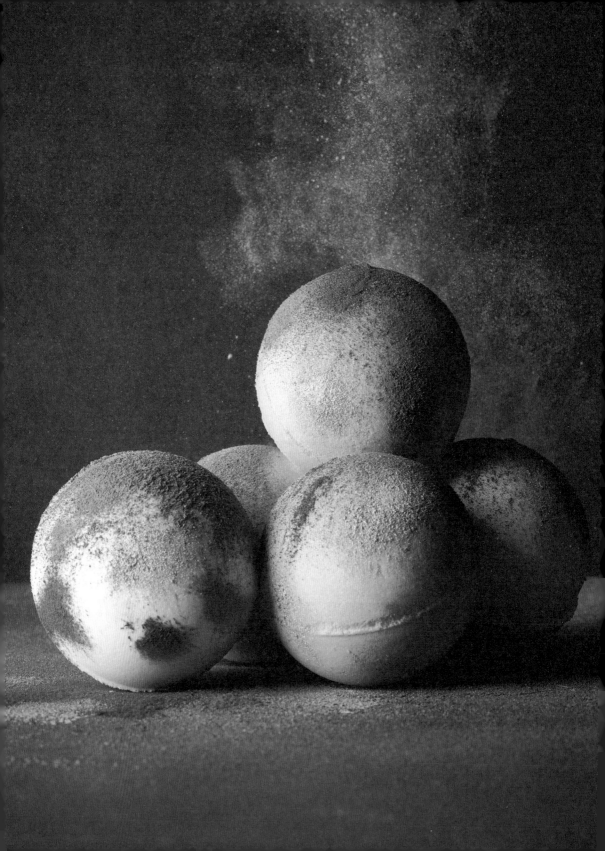

SOMETIMES PEOPLE GET CONFUSED BY OUR BRAND NAME AND SAY IT INCORRECTLY. IT'S A UNIQUE NAME, SO WE GET IT, BUT IT STILL MAKES US LAUGH WHEN THEY DO THINGS LIKE ADD AN *S* TO "DA BOMB" OR CALL OUR FIZZERS "FIZZLERS" WITH AN *L*. THE NAME OF THIS BERGAMONT-SCENTED BOMB IS OUR LITTLE INSIDE JOKE.

THE
FIZZLER
FOJIZZLER

MAKES
3–4
BOMBS

1 In a large bowl, mix together the baking soda, citric acid, and cornstarch.

2 In a separate bowl, combine the oil, fragrance, and liquid color (optional).

3 Add the wet ingredients to the dry ingredients and mix with your hands until the mixture becomes the consistency of wet sand. (If you don't like to get your hands messy, you can wear rubber gloves for this part.) The more vigorous your mixing style, the better the ingredients will be distributed, so don't be shy. Five minutes of stirring, compressing, and kneading should do the trick.

4 Next, press the mixture firmly into your molds, press the mold halves together, and then let the bombs dry for 24–48 hours.

5 Once they are completely dry, remove them carefully from the molds. If you only have one mold, you can also gently remove the bombs as you make them and lay them out to dry on a flat surface. Try not to touch them until they harden.

6 Cover a dry paintbrush with mica powder, one color at a time, and gently flick the brush head to create the spray effect onto the bombs. Handle with care.

2¼ CUPS (497 G) BAKING SODA

1¼ CUPS (288 G) GRANULAR CITRIC ACID

¼ CUP (24 G) CORNSTARCH

¾ CUP (180 ML) OIL

1 TEASPOON BERGAMONT FRAGRANCE

½ TEASPOON YELLOW LIQUID COLOR (OPTIONAL)

3–4 SPHERE-SHAPED MOLDS

1 TEASPOON EACH OF PURPLE, BLUE, GREEN, RED, AND ORANGE MICA POWDER

FIZZ HAPPENS™

LET'S FACE IT. LIFE CAN BE TOUGH SOMETIMES. AND A GREAT WAY TO ESCAPE IS TO HOP IN THE TUB AND DROWN YOUR SORROWS IN SOME FIZZY FUN WITH THIS CALMING, CHAMOMILE-SCENTED BOMB. BONUS: THIS BOMB WILL TURN YOUR BATHWATER BLACK!

MAKES
5–6
BOMBS

2¼ CUPS (497 G) BAKING SODA

1¼ CUPS (288 G) GRANULAR CITRIC ACID

¼ CUP (24 G) CORNSTARCH

¾ CUP (180 ML) OIL

10 DROPS CHAMOMILE FRAGRANCE

⅛ TEASPOON EACH OF BLACK, RED, ORANGE, YELLOW, GREEN, BLUE, AND PURPLE LIQUID COLOR

5–6 CYLINDER-SHAPED MOLDS

1 Mix together the baking soda, citric acid, and cornstarch, and separate out a quarter of the mix (this will be the black mix).

2 Divide up the remaining mix into six equal parts (for the rainbow).

3 Separately, combine the oil and fragrance, and divide as above, coloring the largest part black, and the six smaller parts red, orange, yellow, green, blue, and purple.

4 Add the oil mixtures to each batch of dry ingredients and combine.

5 Mix each batch separately with your hands until each mixture becomes the consistency of wet sand. Wash and dry your hands between each mixing segment. (If you don't like to get your hands messy, you can wear rubber gloves for this part.) The more vigorous your mixing style, the better the ingredients will be distributed, so don't be shy. Five minutes of stirring, compressing, and kneading should do the trick.

6 Press each layer firmly into the molds, 1 teaspoon at a time (in the order of the rainbow), ending with about a quarter of the mold being filled with black mix. Let the bombs dry for 24–48 hours.

7 Once they are completely dry, remove them carefully from the molds. If you only have one mold, you can also gently remove the bombs as you make them and lay them out to dry on a flat surface. Try not to touch them until they harden.

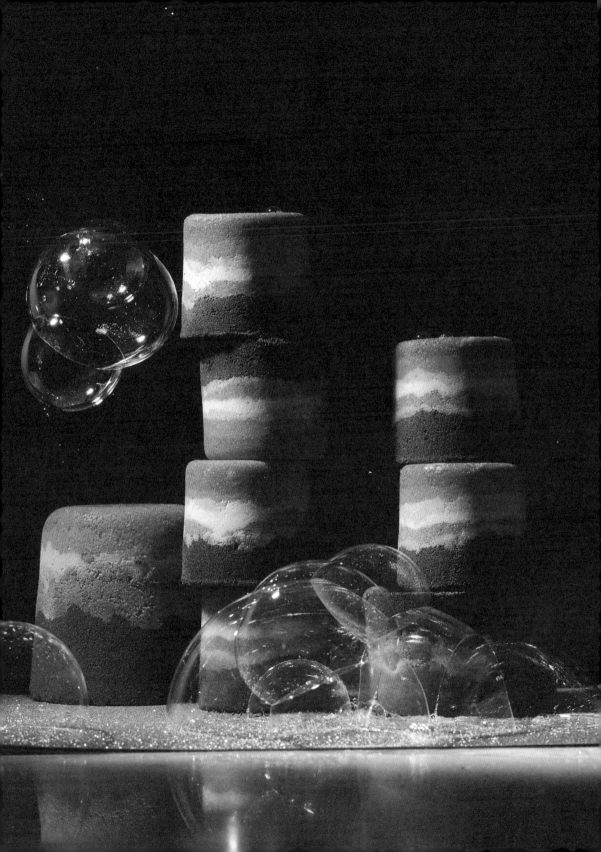

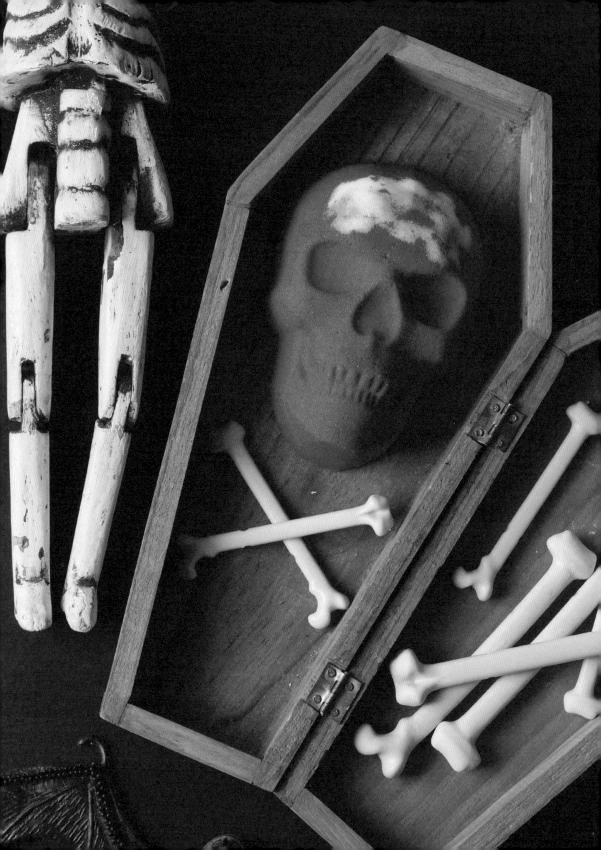

WITCH DOCTOR

HUMANS HAVE ATTEMPTED TO CURE AILMENTS IN A VARIETY OF WAYS, INCLUDING TRADITIONAL HEALING. HENCE, THE TERM "WITCH DOCTOR." THIS IMPOSING, SKULL-SHAPED BOMB CONTAINS WITCH HAZEL, WHOSE SKIN-SOOTHING BENEFITS ARE UNDISPUTED. IT'S KNOWN TO IMPROVE EVERYTHING FROM ACNE AND INFLAMMATION TO ECZEMA.

MAKES 3–4 BOMBS

1 In a large bowl, mix together the baking soda, citric acid, and cornstarch.

2 Set aside a few tablespoons of the dry mix for the skull's forehead section. To moisten this part of the mix, combine it with 1 teaspoon of oil. It is not necessary to add fragrance to this part of the mix.

3 In a separate bowl, combine the oil, fragrance, witch hazel, and liquid color.

4 Add the wet ingredients to the dry ingredients and mix each batch separately with your hands until each mixture becomes the consistency of wet sand. Wash and dry your hands between each mixing segment. (If you don't like to get your hands messy, you can wear rubber gloves for this part.) The more vigorous your mixing style, the better the ingredients will be distributed, so don't be shy. Five minutes of stirring, compressing, and kneading should do the trick.

5 Next, press the mixture firmly into your molds, and then let the bombs dry for 24–48 hours.

6 Once they are completely dry, remove them carefully from the molds. If you only have one mold, you can also gently remove the bombs as you make them and lay them out to dry on a flat surface. Try not to touch them until they harden.

2¼ CUPS (497 G) BAKING SODA

1¼ CUPS (288 G) GRANULAR CITRIC ACID

¼ CUP (24 G) CORNSTARCH

¾ CUP (180 ML) OIL PLUS 1 TEASPOON IN RESERVE (FOR SKULL'S FOREHEAD)

1 TEASPOON EUCALYPTUS FRAGRANCE

2 TABLESPOONS WITCH HAZEL

1 TEASPOON RED LIQUID COLOR

3–4 SKULL-SHAPED MOLDS

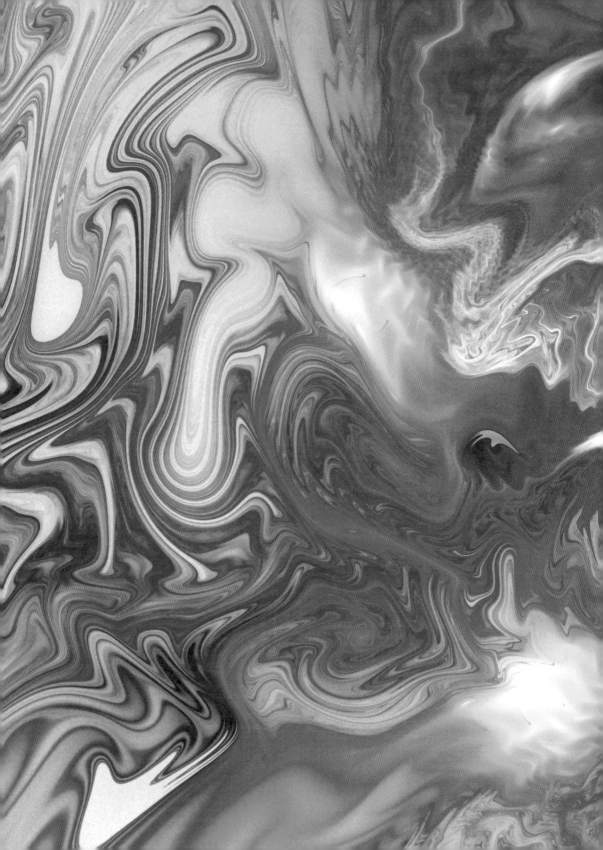

PART TWO

· · · · · · · · · · · · · · ·

MORE BATH + BEAUTY PRODUCTS

FACE, LIPS + HAIR

THE WAY WE SEE IT, SETTING ASIDE A FEW MINUTES A DAY FOR A GLOW-UP IS TIME WELL SPENT. THOUGH WE'VE HAD OUR FAIR SHARE OF "THROW YOUR MOP IN A MESSY BUN AND RUN OUT THE DOOR" MORNINGS, THERE'S NOTHING LIKE A LITTLE PERSONAL GROOMING SESSION TO BOOST ONE'S SELF-ESTEEM.

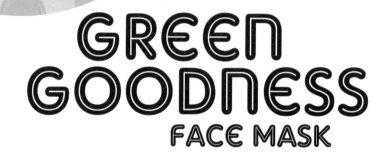

CAROLINE IS OBSESSED WITH AVOCADOS. SHE EATS THEM FOR BREAKFAST, LUNCH, AND DINNER. AND NOW SHE'S FOUND A WAY TO INTEGRATE THEM INTO HER BEAUTY ROUTINE. SEEMS LOGICAL. DON'T FEEL WEIRD ABOUT SMEARING AVOCADO ALL OVER YOUR FACE—IT CONTAINS ALL SORTS OF ANTIOXIDANTS THAT ARE GREAT FOR YOUR SKIN.

MAKES
1
FACE
MASK

GREEN GOODNESS
FACE MASK

½ RIPE AVOCADO

1 TEASPOON APPLE CIDER VINEGAR

1 Clean and dry your face.

2 Mash the avocado and apple cider vinegar together with a fork in a small bowl.

3 Apply the mask to your face and let it sit for 10–15 minutes before washing off with warm water.

YOU'LL BE RED-CARPET READY AFTER USING THIS FACE MASK. IT'S GREAT FOR KEEPING AWAY PIMPLES AND BLEMISHES.

A-LISTER FACE MASK

MAKES 1 FACE MASK

1 Clean and dry your face.

2 Mix the ingredients together in a small bowl.

3 Apply the mask to your face with a cotton swab and let it sit for 10–15 minutes before washing off with warm water.

1 TEASPOON HONEY

1 TEASPOON FRESH LEMON JUICE

2 TEASPOONS PLAIN YOGURT

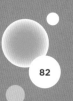

AFTER YOU'RE DONE APPLYING THIS FACE MASK, ADD A BIT OF POMEGRANATE JUICE AND HONEY TO THE REMAINING CHAMOMILE TEA THAT YOU BREWED AND HAVE A CUP!

MAKES 3–5 FACE MASKS

POMEGRANATE POWER FACE MASK

1 BANANA

1 TABLESPOON POMEGRANATE JUICE, SUCH AS POM

1 TABLESPOON HONEY

2 TEASPOONS BREWED CHAMOMILE TEA

1 In a small bowl, mash up the banana with a fork, then mix in the pomegranate juice, honey, and chamomile tea.

2 Apply the mask to your face and let it sit for 10–15 minutes. Keep the remaining mask in the refrigerator.

CAN'T YOU JUST PICTURE YOURSELF RUNNING THROUGH A STRAWBERRY FIELD IN SLOW MOTION WITH A BIG SMILE ON YOUR FACE? THIS FACE SCRUB SMELLS DELICIOUS, AND THE CITRIC ACID IN THE STRAWBERRIES IS GREAT FOR YOUR SKIN.

MAKES
3–4
FACE
SCRUBS

STRAWBERRY FIELDS FACE SCRUB

1 Mash the strawberries with a fork or your fingers, and then mix with the sugar and coconut oil in a small bowl.

2 Let sit for 5 minutes.

3 Rub onto your face in a circular motion, and then wash off with warm water.

4 For more exfoliation, use immediately instead of letting it sit. Keep the remaining scrub in the refrigerator.

3 FRESH STRAWBERRIES

¼ CUP (50 G) GRANULATED SUGAR

1 TABLESPOON COCONUT OIL

UP TOO LATE LAST NIGHT? NO JUDGMENT. GET SELFIE-READY WITH THIS PUFFY-EYE TREATMENT.

MAKES
6–10
EYE
PATCHES

PERFECTION, PLEASE! PUFFY EYE TREATMENT

1 CUCUMBER, PEELED

2 TABLESPOONS WITCH HAZEL

½ CUP (120 ML) ICE-COLD WATER

MASON JAR OR CONTAINER

1 Chop the cucumber into big pieces and then add it to a blender with the witch hazel and water.

2 Puree until well blended and pour into a mason jar or container.

3 To use, dip cotton pads or a small square of paper towel into the mixture and place on your eyes for at least 10 minutes. Keep the remaining cucumber mixture in the refrigerator so that you can refresh the pads when they get warm.

YOU MIGHT THINK OF ROSEWATER AS A WEIRD PERFUME ONLY A GRANDMA COULD LOVE, BUT THIS VERSION MADE WITH REAL ROSE PETALS HAS A LIGHT, BRIGHT AROMA. SPRITZ IT ON YOUR FACE FOR AN INSTANT FACIAL TONER.

MAKES APPROX. 2½ QUARTS (2.4 L)

ROSEWATER REBOOT

1 Add the petals to a large pot and cover with the distilled water.

2 Heat on the stove on medium until the water starts to simmer, then reduce the temperature to low and cover.

3 Continue to cook until the petals have lost most of their color, 20–30 minutes (dark red roses will be a pale pink when done).

4 Let cool, then strain the rosewater to remove the petals.

5 Then add an equal amount of water back into the mixture, place in a spray bottle, and spritz it on your face. We recommend keeping it in the fridge. The mist is even more refreshing when cool!

PETALS FROM 6 ROSES, PREFERABLY ORGANIC

2–3 QUARTS (1.9–2.9 L) DISTILLED WATER

SPRAY BOTTLE

IF THERE'S ONE STEP TO ADD TO YOUR MORNING BEAUTY ROUTINE, CHOOSE THIS ONE. SPRITZ ON SOME SETTING SPRAY AFTER YOU'VE WASHED YOUR FACE BUT BEFORE YOU APPLY YOUR MAKEUP. IT NOT ONLY SMELLS GREAT, BUT IT WILL ALSO TIGHTEN YOUR PORES AND MAKE YOUR MAKEUP LAST LONGER.

MAKES ENOUGH FOR 2–4 APPLICATIONS

LET'S FACE IT SETTING SPRAY

3 TABLESPOONS FILTERED OR DISTILLED WATER

1 TABLESPOON ALOE VERA GEL

1 TABLESPOON WITCH HAZEL

2 DROPS LAVENDER FRAGRANCE

SPRAY BOTTLE

1 Combine all the ingredients in a spray bottle, shake well, and lightly spritz on your face.

2 Keep the remaining spray in the refrigerator, if desired.

BEEN NEGLECTING YOUR SKIN? REDEEM YOURSELF IN AN INSTANT WITH THIS REFRESHING SPRITZ. USE THIS TONER AFTER CLEANSING AND BEFORE MOISTURIZING FOR AN EXTRA BOOST OF VITAMIN C. (WHICH IS AWESOME FOR YOUR SKIN, BY THE WAY.)

MAKES ABOUT 1 CUP (235 ML)

ABOUT-FACE TONER

1 Crush up the vitamin C tablet with a mortar and pestle or the back of a spoon.

2 Pour the powder into a small spray bottle, then add the pineapple juice.

3 Fill the rest of the bottle with water and shake.

4 Mist on your face after cleaning and let dry.

5 Keep the remaining toner in the refrigerator—it feels even better on your face when it's cool!

1 VITAMIN C TABLET, LIKE EMERGEN-C

SPRAY BOTTLE

2 TABLESPOONS PINEAPPLE JUICE

¾–1 CUP (175–235 ML) DISTILLED OR FILTERED WATER

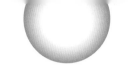

TYPE A AFTERSHAVE STEAMER

STEAM IS GREAT before or after shaving because it helps open your pores. Whether we're talking legs, armpits, chins, or another razor-friendly part, throw one of these steamers in the sink or the shower to maximize the benefits. The energizing eucalyptus and tea tree essential oils will have you ready to seize the day in no time.

MAKES 8–10 STEAMERS

1 CUP (220 G) BAKING SODA

1 CUP (230 G) CITRIC ACID

½ CUP (64 G) CORNSTARCH

½ CUP (120 ML) COCONUT OR SWEET ALMOND OIL

7 DROPS EUCALYPTUS ESSENTIAL OIL OR FRAGRANCE

3 DROPS TEA TREE ESSENTIAL OIL

RECTANGLULAR OR SQUARE MOLDS

1 Mix together the baking soda, citric acid, cornstarch, and coconut oil (or sweet almond oil) until crumbly.

2 Stir in the oils (or fragrances).

3 Press the mixture firmly into the molds, then let dry for 24 hours.

4 Remove carefully. To use, place under hot faucet or throw it in the shower. Once the steaming begins, breathe deeply to take in the wonderful aromas.

ROSEMARY REVIVAL STEAMER

GREAT FOR YOUR FACE, a steamer is like a bath bomb that's placed in the sink. When you run hot water over it, it produces aromatherapy through steam. This steamer uses rosemary, which is good for your skin, hair growth, relieving fatigue, and even aiding digestion!

1 CUP (220 G) BAKING SODA

1 CUP (230 G) CITRIC ACID

½ CUP (48 G) CORNSTARCH

½ CUP (120 ML) COCONUT OR SWEET ALMOND OIL

7 DROPS ROSEMARY ESSENTIAL OIL

3 DROPS LAVENDER ESSENTIAL OIL

¼ CUP (13 G) DRIED ROSEMARY

RECTANGLULAR OR SQUARE MOLDS

MAKES 8–10 STEAMERS

1 Mix together the baking soda, citric acid, cornstarch, and coconut oil (or sweet almond oil) until crumbly.

2 Stir in the essential oils and rosemary.

3 Press the mixture firmly into the molds, then let dry for 24 hours.

4 Remove carefully.

5 To use, place under the hot faucet. Place a towel over your head and lean over the sink, breathing deeply to take in the steam.

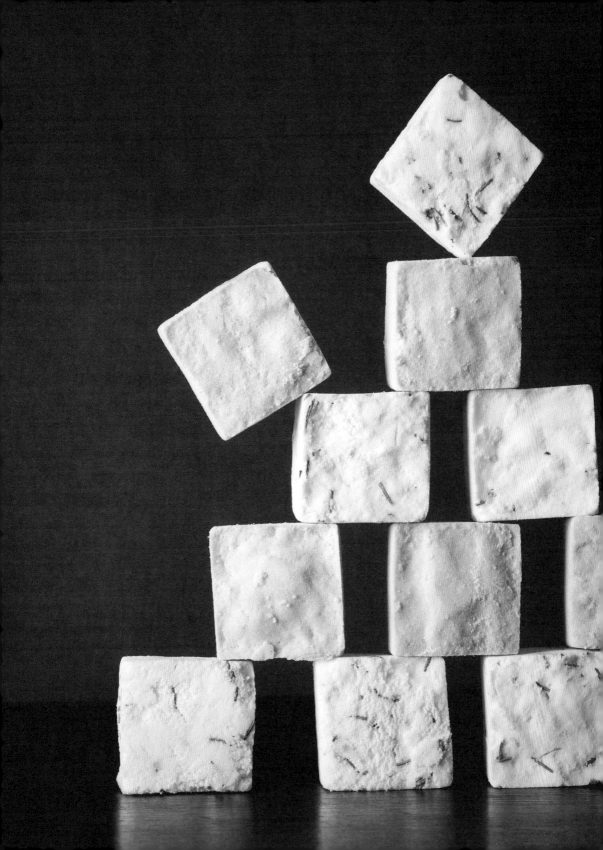

SPARKLE-LIKE-YOU-MEAN-IT
FACE SHIMMER

THIS VERSATILE POWDER will give your face a sparkly shimmer—more mica powder equals more sparkle! (Secret: You can also use it on the rest of your body.)

MAKES 1–2 APPLICATIONS

1–3 TEASPOONS RICE FLOUR

½ TEASPOON ROSE KAOLIN CLAY

¼ TEASPOON MICA POWDER

1 Add the rice flour to the rose kaolin clay until it reaches your desired shade. Mix the ingredients well with a fork, making sure to break up any clumps. Stir in the mica powder. Apply with a makeup brush.

SWEET LIPS
LIP SCRUB

MAKES ENOUGH FOR 2 SCRUBS

DURING COLD WINTERS in the north, our lips can get really dry. When this happens, there's nothing better than a lip scrub and a warm drink to make the corners of our mouths turn upward.

1 TABLESPOON BROWN SUGAR

1 TABLESPOON GRANULATED SUGAR

10 DROPS VITAMIN E OIL

1½ TEASPOONS ALMOND OIL

1 Mix together the ingredients, adding more almond oil if necessary to get the consistency you want (it should be a thick paste).

2 Rub gently over lips until rough patches are gone, then rinse off. To make it easier to apply, use a soft toothbrush. Store any excess in the refrigerator.

YOU CAN USE ANY CLEAN CONTAINER you want for this lip balm with a hint of chocolate and coffee. Try ordering some lip balm tubes online and add custom labels for a perfect gift.

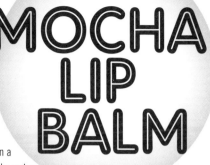

MOCHA LIP BALM

MAKES 10–15 SMALL CONTAINERS OR TUBES

¼ (34G) CUP BEESWAX PELLETS

1½ TABLESPOONS COFFEE BUTTER

½ TABLESPOON COCOA BUTTER (CHOPPED IF NECESSARY)

1 TABLESPOON COCONUT OIL

1 TABLESPOON ALMOND OIL

MASON JAR

15 DROPS VITAMIN E OIL

LIP TUBES OR SMALL CONTAINERS

1 Fill a small saucepan halfway with water and heat over medium heat.

2 Place the beeswax, coffee and cocoa butters, and coconut and almond oils in a mason jar and place the mason jar in the water.

3 Heat, stirring occasionally, until the ingredients are melted together.

4 Add the vitamin E oil and stir to combine.

5 Pour the mixture into containers and transfer to the refrigerator for 20–30 minutes to harden.

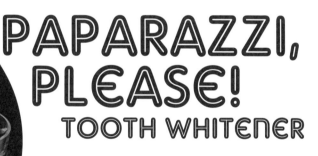

PAPARAZZI, PLEASE!
TOOTH WHITENER

INSTEAD OF SHELLING OUT for tooth whiteners at the store, try this all-natural version to get your teeth smile-ready. (And photo-ready.)

MAKES 1 TOOTH WHITENER

2 STRAWBERRIES

BAKING SODA

1 Mix the ingredients together in a small bowl, then brush onto teeth with a toothbrush.

2 Let sit for 20–30 minutes, then rinse and floss thoroughly.

3 Repeat each day for several weeks to see results.

THIS LIP BALM USES CANDY FLAVORING TO GIVE IT ITS SCENT. YUM!

MAKES 15–20 SMALL CONTAINERS OR TUBES

GIMME LIP LIP BALM

¼ CUP (32 G) BEESWAX PELLETS

1 TABLESPOON MANGO BUTTER

1 TABLESPOON AVOCADO BUTTER

1 TABLESPOON COCONUT OIL

1 TABLESPOON APRICOT OIL

MASON JAR

15 DROPS VITAMIN E OIL

½ TEASPOON CANDY FLAVORING, SUCH AS CHERRY

LIP TUBES OR SMALL CONTAINERS

1 Fill a small saucepan halfway with water and heat over medium heat.

2 Place the beeswax, mango and avocado butters, and coconut and apricot oils in a mason jar and place the mason jar in the water. Heat, stirring occasionally, until the ingredients are melted together.

3 Add the vitamin E oil and candy flavoring and stir to combine.

4 Pour the mixture into containers and transfer to the refrigerator for 20–30 minutes to harden.

HAIR ZOMBIE

WHEN YOU'RE DYING to get rid of all that built-up residue from your usual hair-care routine, look no further than this innovative hair toner. It'll bring your zombie-fied hair back to life. (And you thought that was impossible.)

¼ CUP (60 ML) APPLE CIDER VINEGAR

½ CUP (120 ML) FILTERED WATER

3 MINT LEAVES

AIRTIGHT CONTAINER

1 Heat the ingredients in a small saucepan over low heat. Once it starts simmering, turn it off and let it cool.

2 Then transfer the mixture to an airtight container and place in the refrigerator overnight.

3 The next day, remove the mint leaves.

4 To use, massage into your dry scalp and hair and let it sit for an hour before washing your hair as usual.

MAKES ENOUGH FOR 1–2 USES

MAKES ENOUGH FOR 5–8 USES

GET MISTY HAIR MIST

GOING OUT? A few spritzes of this hair mist will freshen up your hair and give it a bit of *je ne sais quoi*.

3 TABLESPOONS LEMON JUICE

1 TABLESPOON APPLE CIDER VINEGAR

¼ CUP (60 ML) WATER

5 DROPS LAVENDER ESSENTIAL OIL OR FRAGRANCE OIL

SPRAY BOTTLE

1 Combine the ingredients and add to a spray bottle.

DOUBLE DARE HAIR MASK

MAKES ENOUGH FOR 1–2 HAIR MASKS

YOU MIGHT NEED TO WORK UP some courage to put this mayo-based hair mask on your tresses. But if you're up for it, you'll love the results! Mayo is actually perfect for moisturizing your hair because it has protein and oil, which strengthen hair.

½ CUP (115 G) MAYONNAISE

2 DROPS VITAMIN E OIL

1–2 DROPS TEA TREE ESSENTIAL OIL

1 Mix the ingredients together in a small bowl.

2 After washing your hair, apply to wet hair, starting at the roots and working your way through to the ends. Let sit for 15–20 minutes, then rinse out. Keep any remaining hair mask in the refrigerator.

PUMP IT UP VOLUMIZING HAIR MASK

MAKES ENOUGH FOR 1 HAIR MASK

THIS MASK IS A PROTEIN FEAST for your hair, keeping it healthy and thick.

2 EGGS

¼ CUP (58 G) YOGURT

2 TEASPOONS LEMON JUICE

1 TEASPOON LEMON EXTRACT

2 TEASPOONS OLIVE OIL

1 Mix the ingredients together in a small bowl.

2 After washing your hair, apply to wet hair, starting at the roots and working your way through to the ends. Let sit for 15–20 minutes, then rinse out.

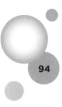

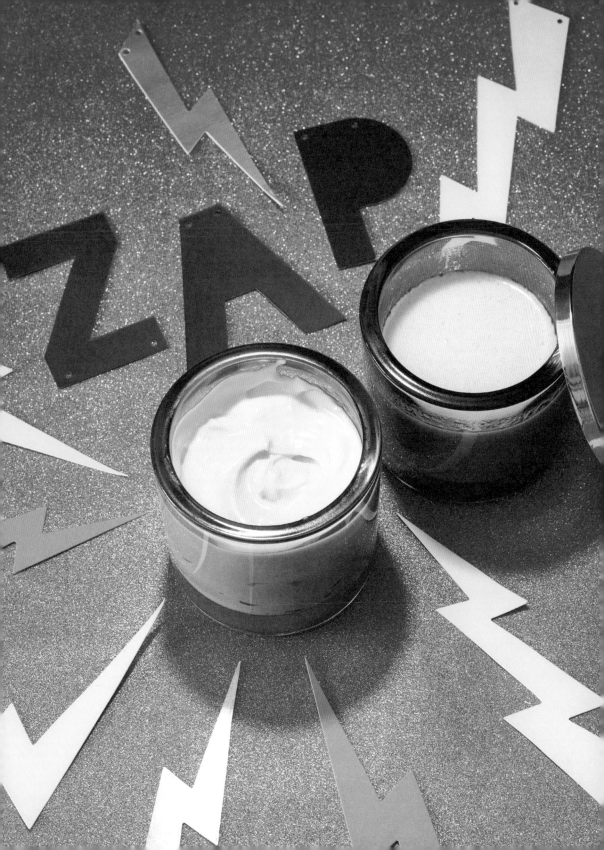

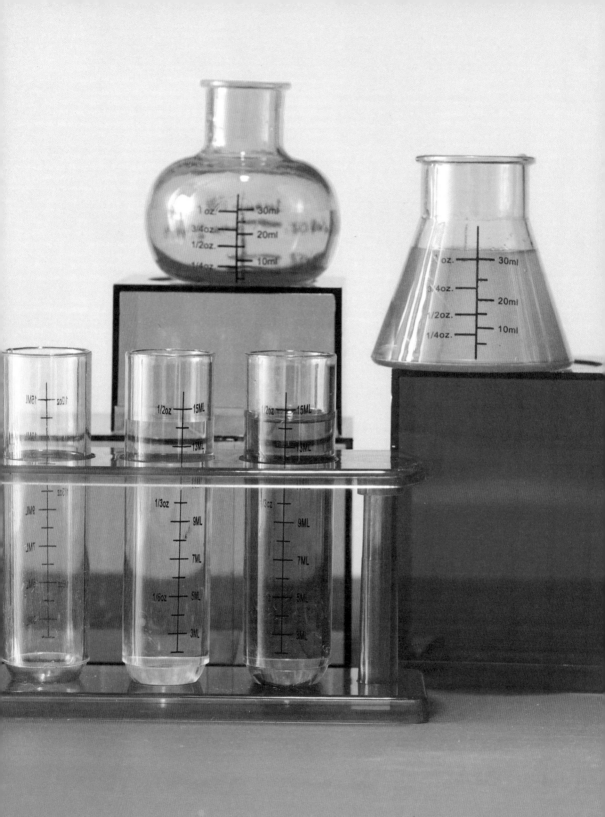

TOTAL HOTTIE
HOT OIL HAIR TREATMENT

THIS HOT OIL TREATMENT is just as good as its salon counterpart, and it's fun and easy to do with a friend when you're having a do-it-yourself spa day.

2 TABLESPOONS COCONUT OIL

1 TABLESPOON OLIVE OIL

MASON JAR

1 Wash your hair.

2 Fill a small saucepan halfway with water and heat over medium heat.

3 Add the oils to a mason jar and place the mason jar in the saucepan.

4 Heat, stirring occasionally, until the oil is warm but not hot.

5 When it's cool enough to touch, massage the oil through your wet hair, starting from your scalp and going to the ends. Work in small sections to thoroughly saturate your hair with the oil.

6 Cover it with a shower cap or towel and let sit for 30 minutes, then wash out.

CURLY Q
CONDITIONING SPRAY

THIS ALL-NATURAL leave-in conditioner will give you bouncy curls and minimize frizz. Plus, it smells wonderful.

¼ CUP (60 ML) FILTERED OR DISTILLED WATER

1 TABLESPOON WITCH HAZEL

2 TABLESPOONS FRACTIONATED COCONUT OIL

1 TEASPOON COCONUT EXTRACT

5 DROPS VITAMIN E OIL

SPRAY BOTTLE

1 Mix together in a spray bottle.

2 Use as a leave-in conditioner or styling mousse by spraying onto damp or dry hair and working it with your fingers.

SOAKS + MELTS

CONSIDER THIS SECTION BATH TREATS 2.0.
HERE YOU'LL FIND SOME FUN, FRESH IDEAS
FOR KEEPING THINGS INTERESTING
DURING TUB TIME, AS WELL AS SOME
SHOWER-FRIENDLY VARIATIONS ON THE
CLASSIC BATH BOMB.

MAKES
3–4
BARS

BEST EVER
BUBBLES BOMB

2¼ CUPS (497 G) BAKING SODA

1¼ CUPS (288 G) GRANULAR CITRIC ACID

¼ CUP (24 G) CORNSTARCH

½ TEASPOON SLES POWDER (SEE PAGE 11)

½ CUP (120 ML) CANOLA, COCONUT, SWEET ALMOND (OUR FAVORITE), OR OTHER OIL

1 TEASPOON FRAGRANCE OIL OR ESSENTIAL OIL

½ TEASPOON LIQUID COLOR (SEE PAGE 10)

3–4 BAR-SHAPED MOLDS

1 In a large bowl, mix together the baking soda, citric acid, cornstarch, and SLES powder.

2 In a separate bowl, combine the oil, fragrance, or essential oil, and liquid color.

3 Add the wet ingredients to the dry ingredients and mix with your hands until the mixture becomes the consistency of wet sand. (If you don't like to get your hands messy, you can wear rubber gloves for this part.) The more vigorous your mixing style, the better the ingredients will be distributed, so don't be shy. Five minutes of stirring, compressing, and kneading should do the trick.

4 Next, press the mixture firmly into your molds and then let dry for 24–48 hours.

5 Once the bubble bars are completely dry, remove them carefully from the molds. If you only have one mold, you can also gently remove the bars as you make them and lay them out to dry on a flat surface. Try not to touch them until they harden.

6 Once they're ready, hold them under a faucet while running a bath.

BATH JELLY IS JUST WHAT IT SOUNDS LIKE—A JIGGLY, JELL-O-LIKE SUBSTANCE THAT MAKES BUBBLES WHEN DROPPED INTO YOUR BATHWATER. YOU CAN CUT THEM INTO SMALL CUBES AND PRESS THEM INTO A LOOFAH IF YOU WANT A PRODUCT THAT EXFOLIATES.

BODACIOUS BATH JELLIES

MAKES 2–5 BATH JELLIES

1 Heat the water in a microwave-safe bowl or glass measuring cup until boiling.

2 Sprinkle the gelatin over the top, stirring carefully so it doesn't clump. Once it's dissolved, stir in the remaining ingredients.

3 Pour the mixture into the molds and refrigerate overnight.

4 To use, hold under a faucet, use like bar soap, or place on the bottom of the shower away from your feet (as the jellies can get slippery), and allow them to slowly dissolve and fill the shower with their fragrance.

⅔ CUP (160 ML) WATER

ONE 7-GRAM PACKAGE GELATIN

4–5 DROPS LIQUID COLORING OF YOUR CHOICE

½ CUP (120 ML) CLEAR BODY WASH, HAND SOAP, OR CLEAR SOAP BASE

2–4 DROPS FRAGRANCE OIL
(IF USING SOAP BASE)

STAR-SHAPED MOLDS

THESE BATH JELLIES
WILL TURN YOUR BATH INTO
A WILD PARTY FEATURING
BUBBLES AND SHIMMER.
(THERE SEEMS TO BE A
RECURRING THEME HERE.)

MAKES
2–5 BATH
JELLIES

GLITTERAMA
BATH JELLIES

⅔ CUP (160 ML) WATER

ONE 7-GRAM PACKAGE GELATIN

4–5 DROPS LIQUID COLORING OF YOUR CHOICE

½ CUP (120 ML) CLEAR BODY WASH,
HAND SOAP, OR CLEAR SOAP BASE

2–4 DROPS FRAGRANCE OIL
(IF USING SOAP BASE)

HEART-SHAPED MOLDS

2 TEASPOONS ECO GLITTER OR
MICA POWDER

1 Heat the water in a microwave-safe bowl or glass measuring cup until boiling.

2 Sprinkle the gelatin over the top, stirring carefully so it doesn't clump. Once it's dissolved, stir in the liquid color, body wash, and fragrance.

3 Pour the mixture into the molds and refrigerate overnight.

4 Sprinkle the glitter or mica powder on top.

5 To use, hold under a faucet, use like bar soap, or lay on the bottom of the shower away from your feet (as the jellies can get slippery), and allow them to slowly dissolve and fill the shower with their fragrance.

LOW-KEY
BATH SOAK

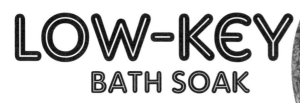

SOMETIMES YOU WANT TO KEEP THINGS REALLY SIMPLE. Here's an easy bath soak made from essential oils and Epson salts.

2 DROPS LEMON OR GRAPEFRUIT ESSENTIAL OIL

2 DROPS ORANGE ESSENTIAL OIL OR FRAGRANCE OIL

2 DROPS BERGAMOT ESSENTIAL OIL OR FRAGRANCE OIL

1 CUP (128 G) EPSOM SALTS

1 Mix the oils into the Epsom salts.

2 To use, add ¼ cup (32 G) of salts to a warm bath under running water.

MAKES ENOUGH FOR 4 BATHS

MILKY WAY
BATH MILK

THIS VANILLA-SCENTED BATH MILK is otherworldly. It saturates your skin with nourishing vitamins and proteins, making it feel incredibly soft.

5 DROPS FRAGRANCE OF YOUR CHOICE

½ TEASPOON VANILLA EXTRACT

10 DROPS VITAMIN E OIL

¾ CUP (167 G) POWDERED WHOLE MILK

¼ CUP (32 G) BAKING SODA

AIRTIGHT CONTAINER (OPTIONAL)

1 Add the ingredients one at a time to a warm bath under running water. Or, if making the bath milk ahead of time, mix well and store in an airtight container.

MAKES ENOUGH FOR 1 BATH

WE ALL MAKE MISTAKES NOW AND THEN. ONCE ISABEL GOT SO CRISPY FROM THE SUN, SHE EARNED THE NICKNAME "LOBSTER LADY." THAT'S A MISTAKE MOST PEOPLE ONLY MAKE ONCE! BUT IF YOU HAPPEN TO OVERDO IT IN THE SUN, THIS BATH SOAK WILL COME TO YOUR RESCUE. IT CONTAINS APPLE CIDER VINEGAR, WHICH IS GREAT FOR SOOTHING AND DETOXIFYING SUNBURNED SKIN.

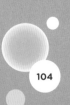

MAKES ENOUGH FOR 1 BATH

OVER-EXPOSED!
SUNBURN-SOOTHING BATH SOAK

½ CUP (120 ML) APPLE CIDER VINEGAR

6–8 DROPS ROSE ESSENTIAL OIL

3–5 DROPS SANDALWOOD ESSENTIAL OIL

1 Add the ingredients one at a time to a warm bath under running water. Soak in the bath for 30 minutes to help a sunburn.

GREEN TEA IS GREAT FOR YOUR SKIN AND IT'S REALLY EASY TO ADD TO YOUR BATH. WE LIKE TO INCLUDE ORANGE PEELS FOR THEIR DISTINCTIVE OILS AND FRAGRANCE, BUT YOU CAN ALSO ADD DRIED FLOWERS OR ANYTHING ELSE THAT STRIKES YOU.

MAKES ENOUGH FOR 1 BATH

TEA TIME BATH SACHET

1 Place the tea bag and orange peel in a sachet or cheesecloth and place under the faucet while running a bath.

1 GREEN TEA BAG
PEEL OF ¼ ORANGE

IT ONLY TAKES A FEW MINUTES TO TRANSFORM REGULAR GEL SOAP INTO SOMETHING THAT'S REALLY UNIQUE, EXCITING, AND . . . WE ADMIT IT . . . A BIT FREAKY! SOME OF OUR EARLIEST MEMORIES INVOLVE SCARING THE HECK OUT OF UNSUSPECTING FAMILY MEMBERS BY SNEAKING INTO THE BATHROOM AND THROWING A BIG BLOB OF THIS STUFF INTO THE TUB.

MAKES
1/2 CUP
(120 ML)
SLIME

THE CREATURE FROM THE CLAW-FOOT BATH SLIME

½ CUP (120 ML) CLEAR SHOWER GEL, LIQUID HAND SOAP, OR CLEAR SOAP BASE

4–5 DROPS LIQUID COLORING

3–4 DROPS FRAGRANCE OIL, IF USING SOAP BASE

¾–1 TEASPOON XANTHAN GUM

1 In a microwave-safe container, the heat the shower gel for 15 seconds on high.

2 Stir gently, trying not to let it bubble too much, and heat for another 15 seconds. Stir.

3 Repeat until the soap is warm.

4 Stir in the coloring and fragrance oil.

5 Sprinkle the xanthan gum over the top of the container and slowly stir in. Continue sprinkling and stirring until the slime is the consistency you want. Make a few different batches in different colors and go wild!

IF YOU TAKE SHOWERS MORE THAN BATHS, YOU'LL LOVE THIS MELT. IT'S BASICALLY A BATH BOMB THAT GOES ON THE FLOOR OF THE SHOWER AND DISSOLVES AS THE WATER HITS IT, RELEASING A BOLD BURST OF FRAGRANCE.

SPRING FLING
SHOWER MELT

MAKES 8–10 SHOWER MELTS

1 Mix together the baking soda, citric acid, and cornstarch in a bowl and divide into three parts.

2 Combine the coconut oil (or sweet almond oil) and essential oils and divide into three parts.

3 Add one color per part to the wet ingredients. Add the wet ingredients to the dry ingredients and mix each batch separately with your hands until each mixture becomes the consistency of wet sand. Wash and dry your hands between each mixing segment. (If you don't like to get your hands messy, you can wear rubber gloves for this part.) The more vigorous your mixing style, the better the ingredients will be distributed, so don't be shy. Five minutes of stirring, compressing, and kneading should do the trick.

4 Press the mixture firmly into the molds, starting with yellow, then pink, then green to create the effect of a pink flower with a yellow center and a green background. Let dry for 24 hours.

5 Once they are completely dry, remove them carefully from the molds. If you only have one mold, you can also gently remove the shower melts as you make them and lay them out to dry on a flat surface. Try not to touch them until they harden.

6 To use, place under a hot shower stream.

1 CUP (220 G) BAKING SODA

1 CUP (230 G) CITRIC ACID

½ CUP (64 G) CORNSTARCH

½ CUP (120 ML) COCONUT OR SWEET ALMOND OIL

7 DROPS LAVENDER ESSENTIAL OIL

3 DROPS YLANG-YLANG ESSENTIAL OIL

¼ TEASPOON EACH OF YELLOW, PINK, AND GREEN LIQUID COLOR

6–8 HALF-SPHERE MOLDS

**MAKES
8–10
SHOWER
MELTS**

COLD
CLOBBERER
SHOWER MELT

1 CUP (220 G) BAKING SODA

1 CUP (230 G) CITRIC ACID

½ CUP (64 G) CORNSTARCH

½ CUP (120 ML) COCONUT OR
SWEET ALMOND OIL

6 DROPS EUCALYPTUS ESSENTIAL OIL

4 DROPS PEPPERMINT ESSENTIAL OIL

¼ TEASPOON EACH OF DARK BLUE,
LIGHT BLUE, AND GREEN LIQUID COLOR

8–10 HALF-SPHERE MOLDS

1   Mix together the baking soda, citric acid, and cornstarch in a bowl and divide into three parts.

2   Combine the coconut oil (or sweet almond oil) and essential oils and divide into three parts.

3   Add one color per part to the wet ingredients. Add the wet ingredients to the dry ingredients and mix each batch separately with your hands until each mixture becomes the consistency of wet sand. Wash and dry your hands between each mixing segment. (If you don't like to get your hands messy, you can wear rubber gloves for this part.) The more vigorous your mixing style, the better the ingredients will be distributed, so don't be shy. Five minutes of stirring, compressing, and kneading should do the trick.

4   Sprinkle all three colors into the molds and stir with a spoon handle to create a swirl effect.

5   Press firmly and let dry for 24 hours.

6   Once they are completely dry, remove them carefully from the molds. If you only have one mold, you can also gently remove the shower melts as you make them and lay them out to dry on a flat surface. Try not to touch them until they harden.

7   To use, place under a hot shower stream.

THIS SHOWER MELT WITH THE SUCCULENT SWEETNESS OF TANGERINE AND THE EYE-OPENING ZAP OF GINGER IS THE PERFECT WAKE-UP CALL AS YOU STEP INTO YOUR MORNING SHOWER.

TANGERINE ZING
SHOWER MELT

MAKES 8-10 SHOWER MELTS

1 Mix together the baking soda, citric acid, and cornstarch in a bowl and divide into two parts.

2 Mix together the coconut oil (or sweet almond oil) and essential oil and divide into two parts.

3 Add one color per part to the wet ingredients. Add the wet ingredients to the dry ingredients and mix each batch separately with your hands until each mixture becomes the consistency of wet sand. Wash and dry your hands between each mixing segment. (If you don't like to get your hands messy, you can wear rubber gloves for this part.) The more vigorous your mixing style, the better the ingredients will be distributed, so don't be shy. Five minutes of stirring, compressing, and kneading should do the trick.

4 Sprinkle both colors into the molds.

5 Press firmly and let dry for 24 hours.

6 Once they are completely dry, remove them carefully from the molds. If you only have one mold, you can also gently remove the shower melts as you make them and lay them out to dry on a flat surface. Try not to touch them until they harden.

7 To use, place under a hot shower stream.

1 CUP (220 G) BAKING SODA

1 CUP (230 G) CITRIC ACID

½ CUP (64 G) CORNSTARCH

½ CUP (120 ML) COCONUT OR SWEET ALMOND OIL

10 DROPS TANGERINE ESSENTIAL OIL

¼ TEASPOON EACH OF ORANGE AND YELLOW LIQUID COLORS

8–10 HALF-SPHERE MOLDS

HANDS, FEET + EVERYTHING ELSE

WHEN WE TELL YOU WE'RE GOING
TO TAKE CARE OF YOU FROM TOP TO
BOTTOM, WE'RE SERIOUS.

LUSCIOUS LEMONS
BODY SCRUB

MAKES ENOUGH FOR 1 APPLICATION

IF YOU'RE SEEKING A SIMPLY WONDERFUL TREAT FOR YOUR SKIN, THIS ONE'S FOR YOU. JUST SLICE A LEMON IN HALF, SPRINKLE ON SOME SEA SALT, AND YOU HAVE AN EASY-TO-APPLY SCRUB.

1 LEMON

¼ CUP (75 G) SEA SALT

1 Cut the lemon into large wedges.

2 Sprinkle a bit of salt onto each wedge and rub on rough patches like elbows, arms, knees, and heels. Wash off with warm water.

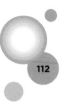

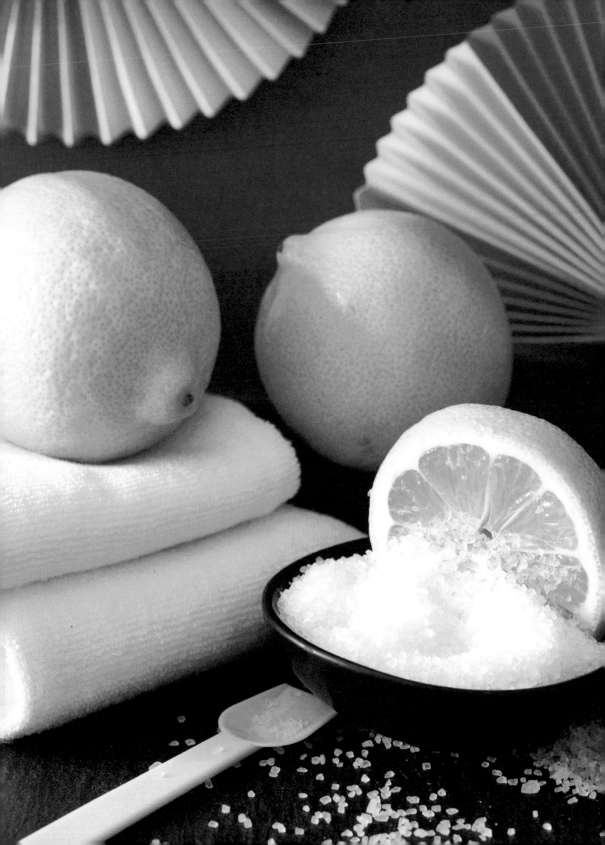

OATS ARE GREAT FOR YOUR SKIN, AND THEY'RE ALSO KNOWN FOR THEIR EXFOLIATING PROPERTIES. IT'S CRAZY HOW SOMETHING THIS SIMPLE CAN MAKE YOUR SKIN FEEL SO SOFT.

MAKES 1–2 SCRUBS

OATMEAL MAGIC BODY SCRUB

½ CUP (40 G) QUICK-COOKING OATS

2 TABLESPOONS SUGAR OR SEA SALT

4–5 TABLESPOONS MILK

1 Grind the oatmeal in a coffee grinder or mash it to break it down. Then add it to a medium bowl with the sugar or sea salt.

2 Stir in enough milk to form a thick paste.

3 Apply the mixture to damp skin using a circular motion, paying special attention to any rough spots.

4 Rinse with warm water. Store any leftover scrub in the refrigerator.

THIS RECIPE IS **GREAT** FOR REMOVING DEAD SKIN. AND IF YOU HAPPEN TO HAVE CELLULITE, YOU'LL BE THRILLED TO HEAR THIS NEWS: COFFEE-BASED SCRUBS CAN REDUCE THE APPEARANCE OF CELLULITE WHEN RUBBED DIRECTLY ONTO ONE'S BUMPY BACKSIDE.

MAKES
1
SCRUB

COFFEE BUZZ
BODY SCRUB

1 Mix together all the ingredients in a small bowl until a damp paste forms (adding more olive oil if needed).

2 Massage over your wet body in the shower using a circular motion, let sit for 5–10 minutes, then rinse with warm water.

¼ CUP (21 G) GROUND COFFEE

2 TABLESPOONS GRANULATED SUGAR

2 TABLESPOONS HONEY

2 TABLESPOONS OLIVE OIL, PLUS MORE AS NEEDED

PUMPKIN PIE
BODY SCRUB

FALL IS A FAVORITE SEASON in our family, so anything pumpkin puts us in a festive mood. This light scrub does wonders for dry, itchy skin and smells good enough to eat. (But please don't. Your skin needs it more.)

MAKES 1 SCRUB

¼ CUP (60 G) BROWN SUGAR

3 TABLESPOONS FRACTIONATED COCONUT OIL

2 TABLESPOONS YOGURT

1 TEASPOON PUMPKIN PIE SPICE

1 Mix together all the ingredients in a small bowl.

2 Massage over your wet body in the shower using a circular motion, let sit for 5–10 minutes, then rinse with warm water.

SPICE UP
YOUR LIFE
HAND SCRUB

WANNA BE CLASS PRESIDENT? Or make homecoming court? This hand scrub won't get you either of those things, but we can promise you this: It will make your day slightly more interesting, and it will cover you in a pleasing cloud of warm, vibrant vanilla cinnamon fragrance. You're welcome.

½ CUP (100 G) GRANULATED SUGAR

½ TEASPOON GROUND CINNAMON

½ TEASPOON VANILLA EXTRACT

2 TABLESPOONS OLIVE OIL, PLUS MORE AS NEEDED

1 Mix together the ingredients in a small bowl, adding more olive oil as needed until a paste forms.

2 Rub the mixture into your hands in a circular motion, then let sit for 10–15 seconds before washing off.

MAKES ENOUGH FOR 2 SCRUBS

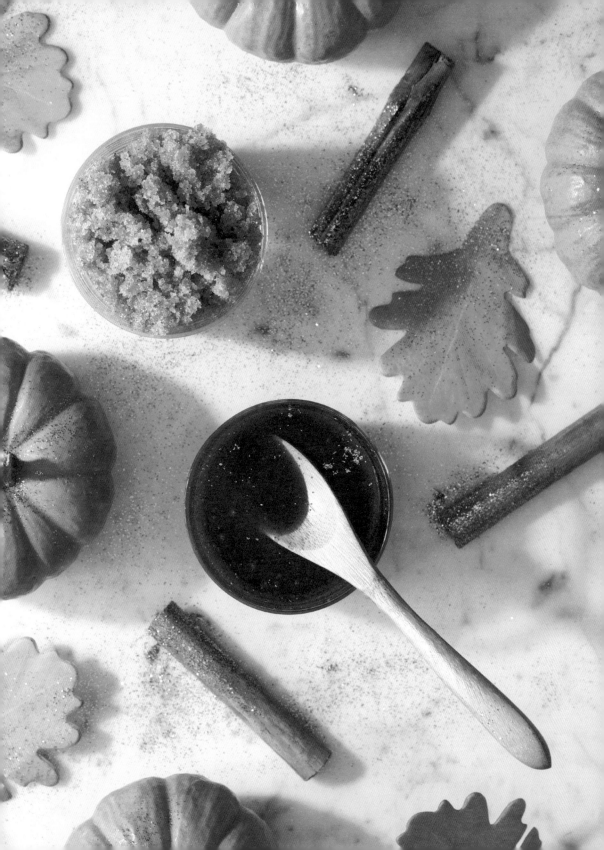

FOR THESE HANDY EXFOLIATING SOAPS, YOU'LL NEED AN ALL-NATURAL LOOFAH (THE STIFF, CYLINDRICAL KIND) AND SOME MOLDS THAT ARE A LITTLE LARGER THAN THE DIAMETER OF THE LOOFAH.

MAKES
3–5
LOOFAH
BARS

SCRUB LIKE YOU MEAN IT
INFUSED LOOFAHS

1 ALL-NATURAL LOOFAH

MOLDS (SLIGHTLY LARGER THAN DIAMETER OF LOOFAH)

WHITE BAR SOAP, SUCH AS DOVE OR IVORY, CHOPPED INTO PIECES

MASON JAR

4–6 DROPS ESSENTIAL OIL OR FRAGRANCE OF YOUR CHOICE

¼ TEASPOON GREEN MICA POWDER

FOOD COLORING, IF DESIRED

1 Using a butcher knife, cut the loofah into slices that are as thick as your molds.

2 Fill a small saucepan halfway with water and heat over medium heat.

3 Place the soap pieces in a mason jar and place the mason jar in the water.

4 Heat, stirring occasionally, until the soap is melted.

5 Add the essential or fragrance oil, mica powder, and food coloring, if using. Stir to combine.

6 Pour the mixture into the molds and add a piece of loofah to each. If desired, place a plate or cutting board on top of them to keep the loofah from floating.

7 Let sit until hardened, 40–60 minutes at room temperature. Once they are completely dry, remove them carefully from the molds. If you only have one mold, you can also gently remove the loofahs as you make them and lay them out to dry on a flat surface. Try not to touch them until they harden.

THESE AROMATHERAPY OILS MOISTURIZE YOUR SKIN AND SMELL WONDERFUL IN THE BATH. YOU CAN ALSO USE THEM AS MASSAGE OILS OR IN LIEU OF LOTION. FOR DIFFERENT AROMAS, TRY SWITCHING OUT THE ESSENTIAL OIL OR FRAGRANCE FOR OTHER COMBINATIONS.

MAKES ENOUGH FOR 8–12 BATHS

ZEN DREAM
BATH AND BODY OILS

1 Place the oils in a container with a lid and mix well.

2 To use, pour a small amount into your hands, then rub on dry spots.

3 To help you fall asleep, rub it somewhere you'll smell it. Or, add a spoonful or two to a warm bath under a running faucet.

¼ CUP (60 ML) AVOCADO OIL

½ CUP (120 ML) COCONUT OIL

3–5 DROPS CEDARWOOD ESSENTIAL OIL OR FRAGRANCE

2 DROPS ORANGE ESSENTIAL OIL

SMALL CONTAINER

IF YOU LOVE THE SMELL OF COCONUT, YOU'LL GO CRAZY FOR THIS EASY DIY HAND CREAM.

MAKES ABOUT ¼ CUP (60 ML) CREAM

CRAZY FOR COCONUT HAND CREAM

¼ CUP (60 ML) AVOCADO BUTTER

1 TABLESPOON FRACTIONATED COCONUT OIL

10 DROPS VITAMIN E OIL

½ TEASPOON PURE COCONUT EXTRACT

SMALL CONTAINER

1   In a bowl, whip the ingredients together with a whisk or fork.

2   Place in a container and use on hands each night.

IF YOU'VE BEEN OVERDOING IT WITH THE POLISH, THIS NAIL SOAK WILL REMOVE STAINS, STRENGTHEN NAILS, AND BRING YOUR FINGERS BACK INTO THE WINNERS CIRCLE.

TOP-TEN NAIL SOAK

ENOUGH FOR 10 FINGERS TO TAKE 1 SOAK

1 Mix all the ingredients together in a bowl, then soak your nails in the mixture for 20–30 minutes.

2 Rinse nails, dry, and apply cuticle cream or lotion.

½ CUP (120 ML) FRESH LEMON JUICE

2 TABLESPOONS WITCH HAZEL

2 TEASPOONS OLIVE OIL

¼ TEASPOON MUSTARD

WHATEVER YOUR GAME, WHATEVER YOUR SPORT, THESE LOTION BARS WILL HAVE YOUR BODY PARTS COMPETING FOR WHICH ONE GETS TO BE PLAYER NUMBER ONE.

MAKES 2–4 BARS

GAME-DAY
LOTION BARS

3 TABLESPOONS BEESWAX PELLETS

3 TABLESPOONS COCOA BUTTER (CHOPPED IF NECESSARY)

3 TABLESPOONS FRACTIONATED COCONUT OIL

MASON JAR

8 DROPS VITAMIN E OIL

30–40 DROPS ESSENTIAL OIL OR FRAGRANCE OF YOUR CHOOSING

BAR-SHAPED MOLDS

1   Fill a small saucepan halfway with water and heat over medium heat.

2   Place the beeswax, cocoa butter, and fractionated coconut oil in a mason jar and place the mason jar in the water. Cover.

3   Heat, stirring occasionally, until the ingredients are melted together.

4   Add the vitamin E oil and essential oil (or fragrance) and stir to combine.

5   Pour the mixture into the molds and transfer to the refrigerator for 20–30 minutes to harden. Remove them carefully from the molds.

IF YOU'RE HEADED INTO THE GREAT OUTDOORS, SHOWER WITH ONE OF THESE MOISTURIZING ESSENTIAL OIL-INFUSED BARS BEFOREHAND. LEMON, THYME, AND EUCALYPTUS ARE NATURAL INSECT DETERRENTS, BUT HUMANS WILL BE DRAWN TO YOUR FRESH, CLEAN AROMA.

MAKES 2–4 BARS

BUG OFF
INSECT REPELLENT BAR

1 Fill a small saucepan halfway with water and heat over medium heat.

2 Place the beeswax, cocoa butter, and coconut oils in a mason jar and place the mason jar in the water. Cover.

3 Heat, stirring occasionally, until the ingredients are melted together.

4 Add the vitamin E oil, essential (or fragrances), thyme, and lemon zest and stir to combine.

5 Pour into the molds and transfer to the refrigerator for 20–30 minutes to harden. Remove them carefully from the molds. Use within a few weeks.

3 TABLESPOONS BEESWAX PELLETS

3 TABLESPOONS COCOA BUTTER (CHOPPED IF NECESSARY)

3 TABLESPOONS COCONUT OIL

MASON JAR

8 DROPS VITAMIN E OIL

5 DROPS LEMON ESSENTIAL OIL OR FRAGRANCE

3 DROPS EUCALYPTUS ESSENTIAL OIL OR FRAGRANCE

2 TEASPOONS CHOPPED FRESH THYME

1 TEASPOON LEMON ZEST

BAR-SHAPED MOLDS

THIS FROTHY SHAVING CREAM IS GREAT FOR YOUR SKIN AND IT'S JUST AS REFRESHING AS A COLD TREAT ON A HOT SUMMER DAY.

MAKES ABOUT 2 CUPS (480 ML) OF FOAM

ORANGE CREAMSICLE SHAVE CREAM

½ ORANGE

MASON JAR

¼ CUP (60 ML) FRACTIONATED COCONUT OIL

2 TABLESPOONS ALMOND OIL

¼ CUP (50 G) MANGO BUTTER

1 TEASPOON VITAMIN E OIL

2 DROPS ORANGE ESSENTIAL OIL OR FRAGRANCE

2 TEASPOONS BAKING SODA

¼ TEASPOON VANILLA EXTRACT

1 Peel and juice the orange and add both to a mason jar along with the coconut and almond oils. Then cover it and place it in the refrigerator overnight.

2 The next day, fill a small saucepan halfway with water, place the mason jar in it, then heat over medium heat.

3 Add the mango butter and heat, stirring occasionally, until the ingredients are melted together.

4 Remove the orange peels. Add the vitamin E oil and essential (or fragrance) and stir to combine.

5 Pour the mixture into a medium bowl and add the baking soda and vanilla extract.

6 Stir briskly with a whisk or an electric mixer until foamy.

7 To use, apply to skin and rinse off after shaving. Store extra in an airtight container in the refrigerator.

DANCE ALL NIGHT
MUSCLE CREAM

ONCE CAROLINE HAD SO MUCH FUN at a friend's sleepover that she forgot about the sleeping part. This thick, soothing cream uses ginger and cayenne powder to help ease muscle pain after a night of whooping it up.

¼ CUP (60 ML) FRACTIONATED COCONUT OIL

1 TABLESPOON GROUND CAYENNE PEPPER

2 TEASPOONS GROUND GINGER

¼ CUP (50 G) MANGO BUTTER

1 TABLESPOON BEESWAX PELLETS

MASON JAR

MAKES 2–4 APPLICATIONS

1 Fill a small saucepan halfway with water and heat over medium heat.

2 Place all of the ingredients in a mason jar and place the mason jar in the water.

3 Heat, stirring occasionally, until the ingredients are melted together. Place in a container and let cool.

4 Apply to sore muscles and store covered in the refrigerator between uses.

SWEET DREAMS
PILLOW SPRAY

SPRITZ THIS PILLOW SPRAY on your pillow or other bedding each night to fall asleep more easily and sleep more deeply. It's way more efficient than counting sheep.

½ CUP (120 ML) DISTILLED OR FILTERED WATER

½ TEASPOON RUBBING ALCOHOL

24 DROPS LAVENDER ESSENTIAL OIL

8 DROPS JASMINE OR YLANG-YLANG ESSENTIAL OIL

4 DROPS BERGAMOT ESSENTIAL OIL

SPRAY BOTTLE

MAKES ENOUGH FOR ABOUT 2 WEEKS

1 Mix all the ingredients together and place in a spray bottle.

2 Spray on your pillow before bed each night.

THIS HANDY FOOT MASK ENLISTS THE HELP OF FUZZY SOCKS TO MAKE YOUR FEET INCREDIBLY SOFT. IT REQUIRES A TIME COMMITMENT, BUT YOU'LL BE SO BUSY SNOOZING YOU'LL HARDLY NOTICE.

MAKES ENOUGH FOR 1 OVERNIGHT TREATMENT

NO BIG RUSH
OVERNIGHT FOOT MASK

¼ CUP (60 ML) VEGETABLE OIL

2 DROPS ESSENTIAL OIL OF YOUR CHOICE

1 Just before bed, mix the oils together, then rub the mask all over your feet and place your feet in some socks. Wake up in the morning with brand-new feet.

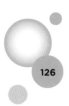

BREAKING IN SOME NEW SHOES? WALKED A FEW TOO MANY MILES? CALM CRANKY PEDS WITH THIS SOOTHING FOOT SOAK.

ANGRY FEET
FOOT SOAK

MAKES ENOUGH FOR 1 FOOT BATH

1 Add all the ingredients to a foot bath or bucket and place your feet inside to soak for 10–20 minutes.

1 GALLON (3.8 L) WARM WATER

4 CHAMOMILE TEA BAGS

½ CUP (64 G) EPSOM SALTS

2 TEASPOONS CHIA OIL

BUCKET (OPTIONAL)

USE THIS SCRUB TO GET GROSS DEAD SKIN OFF YOUR FEET. THE PEPPERMINT ESSENTIAL OIL MAKES THEM SMELL GREAT, TOO!

MAKES ENOUGH FOR 1 APPLICATION

TOOTSIE TINGLE FOOT SCRUB

1 CUP (200 G) GRANULATED SUGAR

2–3 TABLESPOONS COCONUT OIL

2 DROPS PEPPERMINT ESSENTIAL OIL

1 In a small bowl, add the sugar and begin drizzling in the coconut oil until you have a coarse, damp mixture.

2 Stir in the peppermint oil until well blended.

3 To use, rub in a circular motion on the soles of your feet, then rinse off with warm water.

HERE IT IS, OUR LAST BEAUTY PRODUCT! HOPE YOU ENJOYED MAKING THESE AS MUCH AS WE ENJOYED SHARING THEM WITH YOU.

IT'S A WRAP!
FOOT MASK

MAKES ENOUGH FOR 1 APPLICATION

1 Combine the ingredients with a whisk in a casserole dish or washbasin.

2 Place the dish or washbasin on the floor and submerge one foot, then immediately wrap it completely in bubble wrap.

3 Repeat with the other foot. Let sit for 30 minutes before removing the bubble wrap and rinsing your feet.

¾ CUP (175 ML) BUTTERMILK

¼ CUP (60 ML) ALMOND OIL

¼ TEASPOON VANILLA EXTRACT

CASSEROLE DISH OR WASHBASIN

AFTERWORD

SO THERE YOU HAVE IT: enough bath and body recipes to keep you and all your friends buffed, polished, shined, and moisturized well into the next millennium. Once you've had a chance to try out a few of these concoctions, wipe the sweet almond oil off your hands and give yourself a big pat on the back.

Oh, and one more thing. Every good book comes with a fun twist at the end, right? So here it is: We want to see the results of your efforts! Post a photo of something magnificent you made, inspired by this book, and be sure to tag and follow @dabombfizzers, with the hashtag #fizzboombath. We can hardly wait to see what you've been creating!

RESOURCES

AMAZON

When we were first starting out, we purchased a lot of our materials on Amazon.com. Be aware that you're often buying from third-party sellers who control the shipping speed.

BRAMBLEBERRY

Brambleberry.com is the source for all things related to DIY bath products. Find fragrance oils, butters, pigment powders, sodium laureth sulfate, bulk citric acid, and much more.

BULK APOTHECARY

Found online at BulkApothecary.com, this popular website for supplies is great for bulk butters, oils, and other materials and also has a nice selection of fragrance oils.

COSTCO

Costco and other wholesale clubs are a great place to buy large quantities of commonly used items like baking soda and sugar.

LOCAL CO-OPS AND GROCERY STORES

If you have a local co-op grocery store, it can be a great resource for all sorts of raw ingredients. Our local co-op even carries bulk citric acid. You can also try a health-food store like Whole Foods.

MOUNTAIN ROSE HERBS

In addition to having supplies like fragrance oils, MountainRoseHerbs.com has a great selection of containers to put homemade beauty products in.

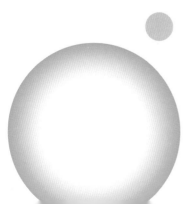

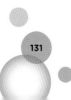

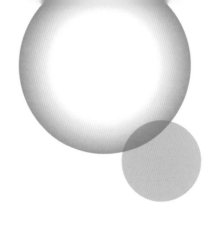

ACKNOWLEDGMENTS

IF YOU LOVE BATH AND BEAUTY PRODUCTS AS MUCH AS WE DO, you can probably imagine how ridiculously excited we were when we were asked to write this book. A wholehearted thank-you to our publisher, Rage Kindelsperger, who gave us this incredible opportunity, taught us something new at every turn, and became a trusted friend along the way.

Thank you to Meredith Harte for your inspired creative direction and to Evi Abeler for bringing magic and life to this book with your astoundingly beautiful photographs. To Chris Krovatin, for keeping the pieces organized and contributing the very best prop of all. And thank you to Jennifer Boudinot for imparting some tremendous wisdom, offering up your stellar bath treat–formulating skills, and also for helping us understand the finer points of writing and editing in Google Docs. And a special thank-you to Mabel LouAnn Harrison for introducing Jen to the world of homemade bath products and for her awesome molds and other supplies.

We'd also like to express our sincere gratitude to Miguel Mozo-Rosario for believing in us enough to become our first full-time employee. We're so happy you did.

To our grandparents, Barb, Ron, Mavis, and Bob, who supported us from the very beginning in endless ways, whether it meant jumping in to package bath bombs each time we had a big order, offering business advice, or unexpectedly giving up Thanksgiving dinner to help us during the holiday rush of 2015. You joined us in the trenches and lived to laugh about it. Most of all, thank you for being our biggest fans.

Next, we'd like to take this opportunity to thank our friends for inspiring us to be our best selves and for putting up with our busier-than-average teen work schedules. A few of you have been there through all the defeats and victories, keeping us supplied with taquitos and frozen coffee beverages in times of need. Grace Lohrding and Kaylyn Schmidt, thank you, thank you, thank you.

ABOUT THE AUTHORS

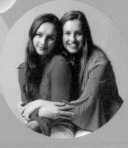

Lastly, sincere thanks to our family, who dropped everything to help us build a company that, little did we know, would change our lives forever. We've learned SO much and always had way more fun than we were supposed to. Thank you to our little brother, Harry. You are wise beyond your years. You're our comic relief and our Smooshie, and is it even legal to be so darn cute? Dad, you're the calm and logic in the moments of chaos. You give us courage to go for our dreams. Lastly, Mom. You inspire us beyond words. Every day you wake up and pour your heart into your work with a level of spirit and creativity that astounds us. Thank you.

We're really happy we got through this without crying. (Not because we're overly emotional, but because we got citric acid in our eyes again. Dang it, that ALWAYS happens.)

WHEN ISABEL AND CAROLINE BERCAW (ages 17 and 16) started making bath bombs in their basement a few years ago, little did they know their hobby would turn into a booming business. Guided by the belief that everyone loves surprises, they created a line of bath fizzers that each have something fun inside. Toys, charms, messages, and jewelry are just a few of the items you'll find inside their products. Since Da Bomb® Bath Fizzers became an official business in April 2015, the teen sisterpreneurs have somehow managed to juggle school and friends, while standing at the helm of a company that has created over 150 jobs in their community. Each fragrant fizzer is handmade in the USA using just a few simple ingredients, and proceeds from the sale of the Earth Bomb go to organizations that clean up the world's oceans.

INDEX

Aromatherapy Fragrances
    Fizz Happens, 72
    The Fizzler Fojizzler, 71
    The Insomniac, 67
    Less Pain, More Gain, 68
    Stress Case, 64
    Witch Doctor, 75

bath bomb how-to, 16–17
body
    Bug Off Insect Repel Bar, 123
    Coffee Buzz Body Scrub, 115
    Dance All Night Muscle Cream, 125
    Game-Day Lotion Bars, 122
    Luscious Lemons Body Scrub, 112
    Oatmeal Magic Body Scrub, 114
    Orange Creamsicle Shave Cream, 124
    Pumpkin Pie Body Scrub, 116
    Scrub Like You Mean It Infused
        Loofahs, 118
    Sweet Dreams Pillow Spray, 125
    Type A Aftershave Steamer, 88
    Zen Dream Bath and Body Oils, 119

cylinder molds
    Candy Crush, 34
    Fizz Happens, 72
    The Insomniac, 67

face
    About-Face Toner, 87
    A-Lister Face Mask, 81

Green Goodness Face Mask, 80
Let's Face It Setting Spray, 86
Perfection, Please! Puffy Eye Treat-
    ment, 84
Pomegranate Power Face Mask, 82
Rosemary Revival Steamer, 88
Rosewater Reboot, 85
Sparkle-Like-You-Mean-It Face
    Shimmer, 90
Strawberry Fields Face Scrub, 83
Type A Aftershave Steamer, 88
feet
    Angry Feet Foot Soak, 127
    It's a Wrap! Foot Mask, 129
    No Big Rush Overnight Foot Mask,
        126
    Tootsie Tingle Foot Scrub, 128
Floral Fragrances
    Color-Changing Birthday Bomb, 61
    Flower Power, 52
    Promposal, 58
    Secret Message Bomb, 55
    Yeah, Baby! Gender-Reveal Bombs,
        56
Fruity Fragrances
    Blueberry Blitzkrieg, 27
    Candy Crush, 34
    The Heartbreaker, 24
    Meet Me in Tahiti, 33
    Strawberry Supernova, 36
    Superstar, 23
    Tangerine Tempter, 31

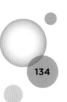

Tiki Time, 30
Zumba Night, 28

hair
  CurlyQ Conditioning Spray, 97
  Double Dare Hair Mask, 94
  Get Misty Hair Mist, 93
  Hair Zombie, 93
  Pump It Up Volumizing Hair Mask,
    94
  Total Hottie Hot Oil Hair Treatment,
    97
half-sphere molds
  Cold Clobberer Shower Melt, 108
  Geode Bomb, 49
  Spring Fling Shower Melt, 107
  Tangerine Zing Shower Melt, 109
hands
  Crazy for Coconut Hand Cream, 120
  Spice Up Your Life Hand Scrub, 116
  Top-Ten Nail Soak, 121
heart-shaped molds
  Glitterama Bath Jellies, 102
  The Heartbreaker, 24

lips
  Gimme Lip Lip Balm, 92
  Mocha Lip Balm, 91
  Sweet Lips Lip Scrub, 90

message bombs
  Promposal, 58
  Secret Message Bomb, 55
  Yeah, Baby! Gender-Reveal Bombs,
    56

Nutty and Spicy Fragrances
  Boyfriend Bomb, 44
  Bronze Goddess, 40
  Cinnamon Twist, 43
  Geode Bomb, 49
  Waffle Bomb, 47

rectangular molds
  Rosemary Revival Steamer, 88
  Type A Aftershave Steamer, 88

skull molds, for Witch Doctor, 75

Soaks and Melts
  Best Ever Bubbles Bomb, 100
  Bodacious Bath Jellies, 101
  Cold Clobberer Shower Melt, 108
  The Creature from the Claw-Foot
    Bath Slime, 106
  Glitterama Bath Jellies, 102
  Low-Key Bath Soak, 103
  Milky Way Bath Milk, 103
  Over-Exposed! Sunburn-Soothing
    Bath Soak, 104
  Spring Fling Shower Melt, 107
  Tangerine Gingerzing Shower Melt,
    109
  Tea Time Bath Sachet, 105
sphere molds
  Blueberry Blitzkrieg, 27
  Boyfriend Bomb, 44
  Bronze Goddess, 40
  Cinnamon Twist, 43
  Color-Changing Birthday Bomb, 61
  The Fizzler Fojizzler, 71
  Less Pain, More Gain, 68
  Meet Me in Tahiti, 33
  Promposal, 58
  Strawberry Supernova, 36
  Stress Case, 64
  Tangerine Tempter, 21
  Yeah, Baby! Gender-Reveal Bombs,
    54
  Zumba Night, 28
square molds
  Flower Power, 50
  Rosemary Revival Steamer, 88
  Type A Aftershave Steamer, 88
star-shaped molds, for Superstar, 23

tiki head-shaped molds, for Tiki Time,
    30
tooth whitener, as Paparazzi, Please!
    Tooth Whitener, 91

waffle-shaped molds, for Waffle
    Bomb, 47

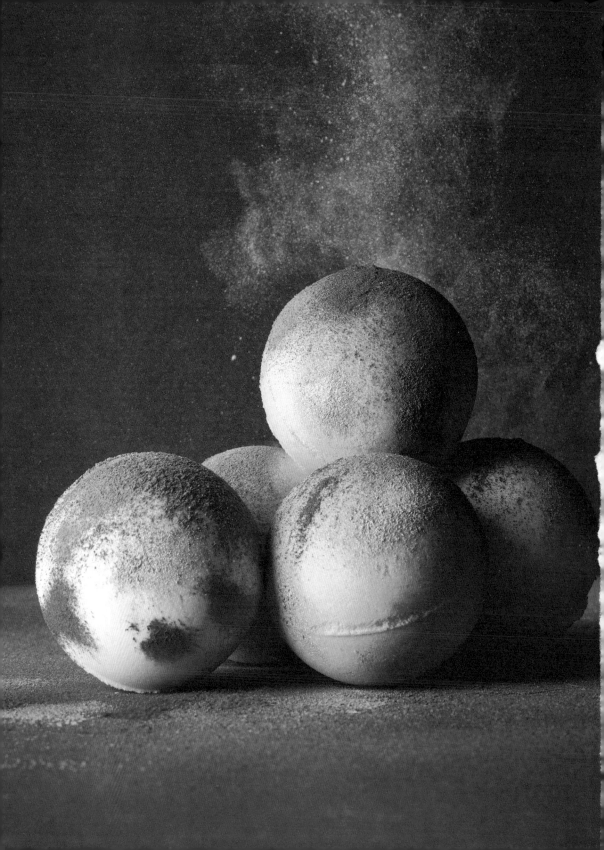